The Healing Power of Echinacea, Goldenseal, and Other Immune System Herbs

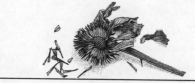

PAUL BERGNER

PRIMA PUBLISHING

ALSO BY PAUL BERGNER

Healing Power of Garlic

Healing Power of Ginseng & the Tonic Herbs

Dedicated to my herbal fathers and grandfathers:
Constantine Rafinesque, Dr. Edwin Hale, Dr. William Cook,
Dr. Eli Jones, Dr. Finley Ellingwood, Dr. Harvey Felter,
John Uri Lloyd, Dr. Henry Lindlahr, Dr. Jesse Shook,
John Lust, Dr. Rudolf Weiss, Dr. Douglas Kirkbride,
Dr. Wade Boyle, and Michael Moore.
May this book increase your rewards.

PRIMA PUBLISHING and colophon are registered trademarks of Prima Communications, Inc.

WARNING—DISCLAIMER: Prima Publishing has designed this book to provide information in regard to the subject matter covered. It is sold with the understanding that the publisher and the author are not liable for the misconception or misuse of information provided. The author and Prima Publishing shall have neither liability nor responsibility to any person or entity with respect to any loss, damage, or injury caused or alleged to be caused directly or indirectly by the information contained in this book. The information presented herein is in no way intended as a substitute for medical counseling.

Library of Congress Cataloging-in-Publication Data
Bergner, Paul.
    Healing power of echinacea and goldenseal and other immune system herbs / by Paul Bergner.
        p.   cm.
    Includes bibliographical references and index.
    ISBN 0-7615-0809-0
    1. Herbs—Therapeutic use.   2. Immune adjuvants.   3. Echinacea (Plants)—Therapeutic use.   4. Hydrastis canadensis—Therapeutic use.   5. Garlic—Therapeutic use.   I. Title.
RM666.H33B47   1997
615'.321—dc21   97–400
                                                                    CIP

97 98 99 00 01 AA 10 9 8 7 6 5 4 3 2 1
Printed in the United States of America

HOW TO ORDER
Single copies may be ordered from Prima Publishing, P.O. Box 1260BK, Rocklin, CA 95677; telephone (916)632-4400. Quantity discounts are available. On your letterhead, include information concerning the intended use of the books and the number of books you wish to purchase.

Visit us online at http://www.primapublishing.com

Contents

ACKNOWLEDGMENTS

I would like to acknowledge the following contributions to this book:

For interviews and personal communications: Mark Blumenthal, Kerry Bone, Howie Brounstein, Richo Cech, Steven Dentali, Steve Gillespie, Feather Jones, David MacLeod, Neil Ray, Herbal Ed Smith, Dr. Jill Stansbury, and Dr. Sharol Tilgner.

For their previous books on echinacea, which I have consulted heavily for this book: Christopher Hobbs and Steven Foster.

For his books on the plants of the mountains, deserts, and canyons of the West, all of which I consulted heavily for information on substitutes for echinacea and goldenseal: Michael Moore.

For his book, *Total Wellness* (Prima Publishing, 1996), which I consulted for information on lifestyle factors that depress the immune system: Dr. Joe Pizzorno.

For research assistance: The Herb Research Foundation.

For patience and editorial assistance: Georgia Hughes and the editors at Prima Publishing.

For inspiration on ecological esthetics: United Plant Savers.

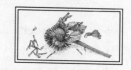

INTRODUCTION

In 1898, Dr. John King of Cincinnati opened a letter containing an unusual request. A Dr. Meyer from Kansas was offering to travel to Cincinnati and let himself be bitten by a rattlesnake in front of Dr. King. He even offered to provide the snake. Meyer would then treat the bite with an herb he called Kansas snakeroot, the use of which he had learned from Native Americans. He claimed to be confident of a safe and speedy recovery.

King was a prominent member of the Eclectic medical profession, a group of M.D.s who, from 1840 until about 1930, used primarily herbal medicines in their practices. Meyer had written to King before, claiming that his "snake root," which we now know as *Echinacea angustifolia*, would cure all manner of infections and poisonings by snakes, spiders, and scorpions. Because of his position of national influence, King probably often received correspondence from flakes or schemers trying to promote quack remedies. He decided to take Meyer seriously, although he did not take him up on the rattlesnake offer.

King and others in the Eclectic profession began experimenting with echinacea, and within twenty years it was the number-one-selling herb in the medical profession. Turn-of-the-century medical books say that doctors used echinacea to treat poisonous bites as well as fevers, cholera, boils, abscesses, chronic ulcers, poison ivy and oak, parasitic infections, acne, nervous headache, meningitis, gangrenous wounds, tonsillitis, respiratory infections, bronchitis, measles, chicken pox, scarlet fever, tetanus, eczema, appendicitis, gonorrhea, and syphilis. Conventional physicians in the U.S. never accepted such claims (and never bothered to research echinacea to any extent themselves), but the same uses of echinacea spread rapidly to Europe, where physicians still use it routinely to treat colds, flu, viruses, and chronic infection.

Earlier in the nineteenth century, the young botanist Constantine Rafinesque traveled through the Ohio and upper Mississippi valleys, studying the native uses of plants. There, he learned of "yellow puccoon," which we know today as goldenseal. Like echinacea, Native Americans used goldenseal for a wide variety of infectious diseases. And, like echinacea, goldenseal became a popular medicine of the Eclectic physicians. They used it to treat infectious diseases of the mucous membranes, digestive tract, urinary and female systems, eyes, and skin. The Eclectics also used goldenseal as a bitter tonic to strengthen a weakened system.

An explanation for how echinacea and goldenseal might act in such a wide variety of conditions had to wait until the discovery of the major components of the immune system. Subsequent scientific research has identified echinacea as an immune system stimulant, and found that constituents of goldenseal will kill bacteria when applied topically.

Echinacea strengthens the body's own antibacterial and antiviral activity, assisting in the fight against virtually any infectious disease. Since the 1950s, about four hundred research papers on echinacea have appeared in the scientific literature, making it one of the most researched herbal medicines in the world. At least three hundred different products containing echinacea are sold in Germany alone, either to physicians or to the general public. Goldenseal stimulates immunity at the level of the mucous membranes, helping the body to kill germs and parasites in chronic infections.

Today, echinacea and goldenseal are among the top-selling consumer-level medicinal herbs in the U.S. They finished first and second, respectively, as the most-prescribed herbs in a 1993 poll of subscribers to my professional *Medical Herbalism* newsletter, just as echinacea did with the Eclectics eighty years ago.

Echinacea and goldenseal are the most famous of the class of *immune system herbs*. Members of this group have been respected as panaceas or cure-alls in different civilizations since early recorded history, though the method of their action was not understood until the recent advances in immunology. Three other important members of this immune system group also appeared among the top medicines in the poll of medical herbalists: ginseng (fifth), garlic (seventh), and astragalus (fifteenth).

In this book, I will describe echinacea, goldenseal, and twenty other immune herbs in detail. I'll explain how to substitute traditional Western herbs, Chinese herbs, Japanese medicinal mushrooms, and other plant substances for often-abused antibiotic drugs. I'll tell you how to treat such conditions as colds and flu, chronic infection, yeast infection, periodontal disease, urinary tract infection, vaginal infection, cancer, AIDS, and autoimmune disorders with herbs, diet, and lifestyle changes.

We are a lot less likely to experience a rattlesnake bite today than we were a hundred years ago. But we still get infections, including new varieties unknown in the past. Dr. Meyer's cure-all herb and its first cousins from around the world are as relevant today to both self-care and professional medicine as they were to the Native Americans and the Eclectic physicians in the last century.

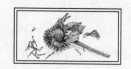

A Note on Conserving Your Health, Your Money, and Endangered Plants

Echinacea and goldenseal are two of the most popular herbal medicines in North America. They are also two of the most often misused plants. If you are like most herb-consuming Americans, you probably know something about them, but you may tend to use them for every situation, even when they are not the most effective herb available. I will explain their appropriate use in this book. If you use them appropriately, you'll probably use them less. I'll also describe more than a dozen other immune-stimulating and antibiotic herbs that are more effective for many conditions.

I hope you'll learn to use these other herbs, not only for your own health, but for the good of the wild plant populations of North America. The growing popularity of echinacea and goldenseal, both in North America and in Europe, is rapidly putting a strain on wild resources. Goldenseal is already extinct in many areas where it once grew freely. The same fate may soon await wild echinacea, which is "strip-mined" by the ton each year in the Midwest. Some of the rarer species of echinacea already face potential extinction at the hands of unethical gatherers.

Part of the threatened extinction is due to loss of natural plant habitat via the development of civilization. There is not much the reader can do about this, but I will ask you to read the sections here on the other immune-system-stimulating herbs. They are less expensive and more effective for some specific conditions than echinacea or goldenseal. And, if you can, purchase cultivated rather than wild-harvested plants or products made from them.

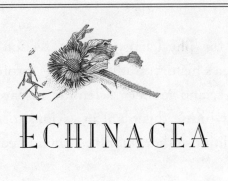

ECHINACEA

ECHINACEA is one of the most popular herbs in the U.S. today. It is best known to the public as a treatment for flu or the common cold, and most people use it in the alcohol-tincture form. Among professional herbalists, it is the number-one herb used in clinical practice, applied to dozens of medical conditions in which weakened immunity or inflammation is a factor. This modern professional use is an echo of the herb's popularity among medical professionals in the early decades of this century. In 1920, echinacea preparations were the best-selling products of the Lloyd Brothers Pharmaceutical company in Cincinnati, Ohio, which specialized in producing high-quality herbal medicines for physicians. In this section, I will cover echinacea's history, traditional uses, professional medical uses, and modern scientific research. You will learn how to use this plant in various forms and for many conditions other than the common cold.

CHAPTER 1

ECHINACEA SPECIES

In North American echinacea products, we find three common species of echinacea: *Echinacea angustifolia, Echinacea pur purea,* and *Echinacea pallida.* Five lesser-known echinacea species usually do not enter into herbal commerce, but are occasionally found in products purported to contain one of the more common species. These three most common species are actually three different medicines. If I simply call them all "echinacea," you will end up completely confused, so throughout this book I'll refer to each species by its proper name. These three species are the most abundant of the wild echinaceas, and the ones used in native and traditional medicine. All three plants have some immune-system-stimulating properties, but they have somewhat different chemical constituents, according to traditional Native American usage, the clinical experience of physicians at the turn of the twentieth century, and the results of modern scientific investigations.

BOX 1.1
THE COMMON NAMES OF
ECHINACEA SPECIES

black sampson	Kansas snakeroot
comb flower	Missouri snakeroot
droops	purple coneflower
hedgehog	scurvy root
indian head	rattlesnake weed
red sunflower	

ECHINACEA ANGUSTIFOLIA

This is the species of echinacea that the Native Americans used "for more purposes than any other medicinal plant," according to one ethnobotanist (Gilmore, 1913). It is also the species that American physicians of the late nineteenth and early twentieth centuries used widely in their practices, treating such severe illnesses as typhoid fever, smallpox, anthrax, blood poisoning, and rattlesnake bite with alcohol extracts of the root. It grows wild in the dry plains from Texas to Canada; east to a line approximately at the eastern borders of Texas, Oklahoma, Kansas, Nebraska, and the Dakotas; and west into the eastern dry plains areas of Colorado, Wyoming, and Montana. *E. angustifolia* is more difficult to cultivate than *E. purpurea,* the more common garden plant which can grow in a wider variety of conditions. Thus, most

E. angustifolia roots available in the marketplace are harvested in the wild.

ECHINACEA PURPUREA

This species is the tallest of the three mentioned so far, sometimes reaching five feet in height. Its leaves are larger than those of *E. angustifolia,* and the lower leaves have small teeth, a characteristic that distinguishes it from the other two species. It is the most common garden species of echinacea, the easiest to grow commercially, and the one that appears most often in American products. There are few Native American uses for *E. purpurea;* the only recorded ones are for coughs, indigestion, and gonorrhea. The Eclectic physicians did not favor *E. purpurea,* but this may have been due to substitution of look-alike roots of other plants for those of *E. purpurea.* Herbalists and physicians today use *E. purpurea* interchangeably with *E. angustifolia* because they have similar clinical properties. Today *E. purpurea* is widely cultivated, and identification is not the problem that it was a century ago.

Most modern scientific research into *E. purpurea* has focused on the leaves and flowers of the blooming plant. Various constituents have been found to be potent immunostimulants in animal and petri dish studies. The history of the use of *E. purpurea* flowering tops goes back to the 1930s, when a German pharmaceutical company attempted to obtain *E. angustifolia* for replanting in Germany and inadvertently purchased *E. purpurea.* The Germans began extensive testing of *E. purpurea* for immune-system-stimulating properties. Rather than using the root, as is the case with *E. angustifolia,* they developed products using the flowering tops of *E. purpurea.* Because echinacea is a perennial, there is an advantage to working with the flowering tops: the stem can be cut off each year to six or eight inches above the ground, and the whole plant will grow back the next year without replanting.

A popular German preparation of the juice of the flowering tops, stabilized with twenty-two percent alcohol, has been sold in Germany since the 1930s. This was the first introduction of *E. purpurea* into common medical usage, and it has been popular ever since. Recent research has found this product to be effective in treating various kinds of infections and inflammations.

ECHINACEA PALLIDA

This species is similar to *E. angustifolia,* but it is taller and its petals droop downward more sharply toward its stem — thus the common name "droops" is applied to this species in some parts of the country. Its main habitat is just to the east of that of *E. angustifolia,* eastward into Arkansas and Missouri, across Illinois to the Indiana border, and north through Iowa and to the southern border of Wisconsin. *E. pallida* was used by the Native Americans to treat infectious diseases and snakebite, but some tribes may have held that *E. angustifolia* was the stronger medicine (Bauer and Wagner, 1990).

Much of the root sold in the U.S. today as *E. angustifolia* is actually *E. pallida,* although the product will probably not say so on the label. The *E. pallida* roots are larger, more dense, and easier to collect than *E. angustifolia.* This adulteration has probably been occurring for more than one hundred years. The Eclectic physicians of the last century, in the botanical descriptions contained in their medical books, often failed to distinguish between *E. pallida* and *E. angustifolia,* apparently not realizing that they were different species.

BOX 1.2
SOME BOTANICAL NAMES FOR
THE *ECHINACEA* GENUS

Sometimes botanists take centuries to agree
on a name for a plant. Below are some of
the botanical names that have been used
for *Echinacea*, the name eventually agreed
upon at an International Botanical Congress
in 1959:

Chrysanthemum americanum
(L. Plunkenett, 1696)

Drancunclus virginanus latifolius (Morrison, 1699)

Rudbeckia purpurea (Linnaeus, 1753)

Brauneria spp. (N.J. de Necker, 1790)

Echinacea purpurea (Conrad Moench, 1794)

Helichroa spp. (Rafinesque, 1830)

The word "echinacea" is derived from the
Greek word "echinos," meaning "hedgehog"
or "sea urchin." This is a reference to the
spiny projections on the seed heads of
the flower, something common to all the
echinacea species.

In the 1931 herbal classic, *A Modern Herbal,* Grieve lists *E. pallida* as a synonym for *E. angustifolia.* Thus, some of the information we have from that era describing *E. angustifolia* probably applies to *E. pallida.* The Eclectic doctors also noted that echinacea was highly variable in its clinical effectiveness, and this variability may have been due to confusing these two roots, possibly also failing to distinguish it from *Parthenium integrifolium,* which I will describe in Chapter 8.

The failure to distinguish between the *angustifolia* and *pallida* species has also plagued modern research. As we will see in Chapter 5, some scientific studies of *E. angustifolia* were probably actually performed on *E. pallida. E. pallida* is considered by most North American herbalists to be an inferior species as a medicine.

LESS WELL-KNOWN AND RARE SPECIES

Five other echinacea species are known to botanists, but do not usually appear in products in North America. For more detail on these species, including how to obtain seed and grow them, see Steven Foster's *Echinacea: Nature's Immune Enhancer* (Foster, 1991). *Echinacea atrorubens* is relatively rare, appearing only in patches in the south central plains. *Echinacea paradoxa* is also rare, occurring naturally only in the Ozark mountains and surrounding areas; it has yellow flowers. *Echinacea sanguinea* is more common than the above two species and grows mostly in eastern Texas and western Louisiana. *Echinacea simulata* closely resembles *E. pallida* and appears in patches in the south central Midwest. Two endangered species—*Echinacea laevigata* and *Echinacea tennesseensis*—grow in Tennessee and states farther to the east.

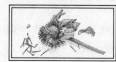

ECHINACEA
IN MEDICAL
HISTORY

The story of the discovery and eventual worldwide fame of echinacea closely follows the evolution of American medicine during the 1800s. Medicine at the time of American independence was almost nothing like what we know as medicine today. Doctors trained in the European model of that time were known as members of the "Regular school." This was a low point in the history of Western medicine, and these doctors practiced bloodletting, violent purging, and the use of extremely poisonous minerals such as mercury. Many people considered a visit to the doctor as the last alternative before visiting the undertaker. The herbs they used, if any, tended to be strong in their action, and potentially poisonous.

At the same time, some European colonists had brought their own medicines with them, and medicinal herb gardens and medical self-care with herbs were part of many households and communities. Dozens of the herbs they brought eventually took up permanent residence here and are native throughout the U.S. today. The settlers also learned the use of many North American plants, including echinacea, from Native Americans. Practitioners known as "Root doctors" or "Indian doctors" used these herbs along with their garden herbs, rather than the stronger methods of the Regulars.

In the first decades after American independence, both lay practitioners and some physicians trained in the Regular school turned to the methods of the Root and Indian doctors. A rebellion against the Regulars paralleled the rebellion against the British, and eventually led to the establishment of various medical "sects" in the U.S. The most important of these sects were Thompsonian herbalism, physiomedicalism, homeopathy, and the Eclectic school. Strife between these sects and with the Regulars characterized the entire nineteenth century and the first decades of the twentieth century.

The Regulars were almost eliminated as a profession during the 1840s after the successes of the rival schools during epidemic disease outbreaks in the Eastern cities. Medicine was deregulated during that time, and the Regulars had no advantage of licensing over the other doctors. It was during this time that the American Medical Association was formed, to protect the interests of the Regulars against the competition that dominated them. From the time of independence right through the decade after World War I, a collective movement by physicians of various schools sought to establish a truly North American method of medicine using native plants.

The Regulars eventually won out, and between 1910 and 1930 used political maneuvering to eliminate the other schools. They became what we call "conventional medicine" today. Ironically, many of the North American plants that were shunned by the American Regular physicians became leading medicines in Europe, even among the Regulars there. Echinacea, condemned by the Regular school in the years after its discovery, is frequently prescribed by M.D.s in Germany today.

Try to imagine what exposure to the new North American plants must have been like for the European colonists, and especially for plant-loving botanists, physicians, and lay healers. They encountered whole new ecosystems rich with plants they had never seen before. This was, to them, the New World—somewhat like a new planet would be for us today. They also encountered an existing civilization here, and the Native Americans often helped them through periods of life-threatening illness by teaching them the medicinal uses of North American plants.

So it was a combination of wonder, curiosity, and love for the new plants—a call for a rational medicine in the face of the medical abuses of the day and a rebellion against the old orthodoxy of medicine—that led to the development of the new schools of medicine here.

EARLY REFERENCES

Although mention of the echinacea plant had occurred in botanical circles before that time (see Box 1.2), the first published mention of echinacea as a medicine appeared in 1762 in *Flora Virginica,* a European book on the botany of the plants of Virginia (Gronovius). That book reflected the work of an English botanist named John Clayton. *E. purpurea* was mentioned as a cure for ulcers on horses' backs caused by saddles. The purpurea species was the first to appear in the literature because its natural habitat is the eastern U.S., the area first colonized by the Europeans. The western angusti-folia and pallida species appeared in the literature later, as the Europeans made closer contact with the Western Native Americans and learned their uses of these plants. This early mention of *E. purpurea* was later cited as a reference in the *Materia Medica Americana*, the first scholarly description of the new American medicinal plants, published in Germany in the first decade after American independence by Johann Schöpf (Schöpf, 1787).

The first mention of medicinal uses of echinacea in humans came from botanist Constantine Rafinesque, in the 1830 version of his botanical classic, *Medical Flora*. Rafinesque was a key figure in the development of the new American plant medicines. Although eccentric as a botanist, with a tendency to give new and unconventional names to plants—echinacea included—his contribution to the discovery and use of American medicinal plants is immeasurable. His botan-ical works and records of native uses of plants became a primary source for the medical books of all the major schools of medicine that followed in the next hundred years. The Regular school cited him, even if they were sometimes critical of his observations.

Rafinesque might also be called one of the founders of the Eclectic school of medicine, whose practitioners used botanical medicines and were prominent in the U.S. from the 1820s until the 1930s. I'll cover this school, and how its doctors used echinacea, in detail in Chapter 3. Rafinesque was the first to coin the term "Eclectic" and to expound the philosophy of the school (Boyle, 1988).

Rafinesque was an explorer. In the first decades of the nineteenth century, he traveled throughout the Ohio and

Mississippi River valleys, studying the plants there, be-friending the Native Americans, and recording native medic-inal uses for plants. These travels remain an extremely important recording of the uses of plants, because they were conducted before the relocation of many of the Eastern and Midwestern tribes.

In was on one of these journeys that Rafinesque en-countered echinacea. Rafinesque called the genus "He-lichroa," rather than using one of the names already existing for it (see Box 1.2) (Bauer and Wagner, 1990). Writers who followed Rafinesque, including the famous Eclectic John King, have erroneously concluded that Rafinesque was re-ferring to *E. purpurea* in his recording of this plant.

Rafinesque referred to the Mandan use of Helichroa for the treatment of syphilis. The Mandan, who spoke a vari-ant of the Sioux language, were an important cultural group in the Northern Plains. Their villages, located at a major river junction in North Dakota, were key trading centers for French trappers. This is the natural range of *E. angustifolia,* and if the Mandan used any species for the treatment of syphilis, it was that one and not *E. purpurea,* which grows far to the south and east of that area. Rafinesque also cites Schöpf's earlier mention of *E. purpurea* for treating the saddle sores of horses. Thus, Rafinesque wrote about the uses of both the angustifolia and the purpurea species, without dis-tinguishing between them.

NATIVE AMERICAN USES

Native American tribes throughout the Great Plains used echinacea, and we can conjecture that peoples of the area have used it for tens of thousands of years. It was via these

Plains Indians that echinacea entered into American professional medicine some fifty years after Rafinesque first
recorded its use. According to the ethnobotanist Gilmore,
echinacea was one of the Native Americans' most important
medicines, being used as a remedy for more conditions than
any other plant (Bauer and Wagner, 1990). Table 2.1, syn-
thesized from several works, shows the native uses of the
three echinacea species (Bauer and Wagner, 1990; Foster,
1991; Hobbs, 1990).

TABLE 2.1   NATIVE USES OF THE THREE
ECHINACEA SPECIES

E. angustifolia

Used by the Cheyenne, Comanche, Crow, Dakota, Kiowa, Montana,
Omaha, Pawnee, Ponce, Teton Sioux, and Winnebago tribes.

Use	Form
Analgesic for sore neck	Tea of leaves and roots rubbed into muscles
Anesthetic	Pulp of pounded roots applied to arms and hands
Inflammation of the mouth, gums, and throat	Tea of leaves and roots or a decoction of the root as a mouthwash or gargle
Inflammation of the eyes	Roots
Toothache	Juice or tea of the roots
Burns, pain relief	Juice
Headache	Smoke therapy
Poison antidote	Internal applications
Mumps	Juice or plant pulp as external application
Snakebite and other poisonous bites and stings	External and internal application
Coughs, colds, and sore throats	Chewed roots

Septic diseases   Chewed roots
Tonsillitis
Hydrophobia
Abdominal complaints
Colic

E. pallida

Used by the Cheyenne, Dakota, and Meskwaki tribes (Fox).

Use	Form
Menstrual cramps and other spasmodic complaints	Roots
Arthritis and rheumatism	Decoction of the roots
Burns	Wash with the tea
Colds	Roots
Toothache	Placed in cavities in teeth
Boils	Roots
Poisoning	Roots
Eye inflammation	Roots
Feverish complaints	Roots
Smallpox	
Measles	
Mumps	
Snakebite	

E. purpurea

Used by the Choctaw and Delaware-Oklahoma tribes.

Use	Form
Cough	Chewing the root
Dyspepsia (indigestion)	
Gonorrhea	

(Source: Bauer and Wagner, 1990; Foster, 1991; Hobbs, 1990)

Ethnobotanical studies show that *E. angustifolia* and *E. pallida* were used by more tribes and for a wider variety of purposes than was *E. purpurea,* for which we have only a handful of recorded uses. There is some opinion that *E. angustifolia* and *E. pallida* were used interchangeably. In an area of the West where both plants may occur, the Omaha Indians distinguished between larger and smaller ("male" and "female") echinaceas, stating that the smaller variety was a more potent medicine. German researchers suggest that the larger plant is *E. pallida,* and *E. angustifolia* the smaller one, and that the distinction could have been between these two species. Foster suggests that the taller variety could be a taller variant of *E. angustifolia* that resembles *E. pallida* (Foster, 1991). Subsequent research has shown that *E. angustifolia* and *E. pallida* have different chemical constituents, and modern herbalists consider *E. pallida* to be of questionable clinical value.

Ethnobotanists do not mention *E. purpurea* much as a medicine, and it was only used to treat a few conditions. This could be for several reasons. First, obviously, is the possibility that the Native Americans did not use it much as a medicine. Another is that most records of Native American uses of plants were made after the Native Americans of the eastern U.S., where *E. purpurea* is native, had been relocated to reservations in the West. *E. purpurea* never figured prominently in early American medicine, and entered into professional medical practice only after the German introduction of a product made from the tops of the purpurea plant in the 1930s.

The native applications of the other echinacea species were quite varied, and many are still in medical use today,

TABLE 2.2   NATIVE AMERICAN NAMES
             FOR ECHINACEA

Fox:	*wetop:* widow's comb
	ashosikwimia'kuk: smells like a muskrat scent
Omaha-Ponca:	*mika-hi:* comb plant
	ikigahai: comb
	inshtogahte-si: eye medicine
Pawnee:	*ksapitahako:* "whirl," from a game children would play by whirling two echinacea stalks around each other
	saparidu kahts: mushroom medicine, referring to the similarity between the echinacea flower head and a mushroom
Dakota:	*ichalipe-hu:* whip plant

either in the U.S. or in Europe. The most common method was to chew the fresh root. The root might also be crushed, and the pulp applied externally to a wound or skin infections. The juice of the root was also drunk or applied externally. Less frequently, a tea was made; the alcohol tincture was unknown among the Native Americans. Mention is also made of "smoke therapy" (Bauer and Wagner, 1990), although it is not clear whether the plant was smoked like tobacco, or whether the smoke was applied externally, both methods being common applications of various plants among the Plains Indians.

THE MID-1800S

Between Rafinesque's writings in 1830 and the introduction of *Echinacea angustifolia* into Eclectic medical practice in the 1880s, spotty mentions of echinacea appear in American medical literature. The first of these, cited by Hobbs, was in a medical journal article appearing in 1847. The author states that "the tincture or decoction is a specific for the venereal disease in its worst forms, having never been perseveringly employed without success." (Comings, 1847). Botanist Asa Gray's *Manual of Botany* (1848) states that *Echinacea purpurea* has a "root thick, black, very pungent to the taste, used in popular medicine under the name black sampson."

In 1852, the fifth year after the founding of the American Medical Association, Clapp mentioned *E. purpurea* in the *Transactions of the American Medical Association*, where he stated that the root was used in popular medicine for indigestion. Finally, John King, one of the giants of the Eclectic medical profession, mentioned *E. purpurea* in his famous *materia medica* (list of medicines) of 1852, using the name *Rudbeckia purpurea*. He stated that it was used with benefit in syphilis. King may have simply been echoing the earlier reference by Rafinesque, in which case the correct plant is *E. angustifolia* rather than the purpurea species.

Dr. F.V. Hayden, in an 1859 report to the government on plants used by the Plains Indians, made the first published mention of echinacea as a treatment for snakebite. He also named the purpurea species, but from his description, it seems that the plant was actually *E. angustifolia* or *E. pallida*. Later in the century, one of the Eclectics claimed that *E. angustifolia* had been unknown in medicine before the mid-1880s (Felter and Lloyd, 1898). Actually that species' uses had been described by Rafinesque, King, and Hayden before that time, but the species was misidentified as *E. purpurea*.

Echinacea as Snake Oil: The Story of Dr. H.C.F. Meyer

Echinacea did not come into widespread use by the medical profession until after 1887, though rumors about it had circulated in medical literature for about a hundred years prior to that date. Echinacea made its transition from Native American panacea to one of the most frequently prescribed medicines in the country through the person of a Dr. H.C.F. Meyer of Pawnee City, Nebraska. Just who Dr. Meyer was, or what his training was, has eluded historians. He has been referred to as a "quack" doctor—a seller of "snake oil" remedies (Foster, 1991)—and as a homeopath (Madaus, 1938). Whatever his background, historians agree that Meyer learned the use of echinacea from the Native Americans, that he mixed it with some other herbs and sold the mixture as a proprietary formula, and that he claimed to have experimented extensively with the use of echinacea for the treatment of rattlesnake bites.

The only detailed account of Meyer's discovery of echinacea comes in a German-language account written almost seventy years after the fact. Thus it may be romanticized. On the other hand, Meyer himself was German—the label on his product was written in both German and English—so it is possible that German sources knew more about his background than did Americans. According to that account:

A homeopathic doctor [Meyer] observed a Native American woman crushing echinacea plants between two stones, and asked her what they were used for. She told him that the plant pulp prepared this way served as a poultice for wounds, that it helped them to heal more quickly, and that it was also good for rattlesnake bites.

(Madaus, 1938)

Meyer apparently began using echinacea—the angustifolia species native to Nebraska—in 1870 without knowing the botanical identity of the plant. He mixed echinacea with at least two other herbs—wormwood and hops—and sold it in a secret formulation as "Meyer's Blood Purifier." After fifteen years of using the mixture on patients, Meyer wrote to the prominent Eclectic professor John King and to pharmacist John Uri Lloyd to get their endorsement of the mixture. He included samples of echinacea plants and tincture and wrote that echinacea was an "antispasmodic and antidote for blood poisoning." He also sent a long list of illnesses that he had "cured" with his product (see Box 2.1). The German-language claims on the label of Meyer's original product are as follows:

Take one ounce three times a day in the following cases: rheumatism, neuralgia, sick headache, erysipelas, dyspepsia, old tumors and ulcers, open wounds, dizziness, scrofula [swollen glands], and sore eyes. In cases of poisoning by plants or other sources, take double the dose. For rattlesnake bite, take a triple dose, which will bring about absolute cure within twenty-four hours. Children under ten should take half the normal dose.

(Lloyd, 1924)

BOX 2.1

DR. MEYER'S CLAIMS OF AILMENTS CURED BY HIS ECHINACEA MIXTURE

acne

bites and stings of bees, wasps, spiders, etc.

boils

carbuncles

cholera morbus

cholera infantum

colic in horses

eczema

erysipelas (skin infection caused by *Staphylococcus* bacterium)

fevers, including typhoid, congestive, and remittent

hemorrhoids

internal abscesses

malarial fever

milk crust

nasal and pharyngeal catarrh

nervous headache

old ulcers

poison ivy and oak

scrofulous ophthalmia

trichinosis

typhoid fever (internal and local to abdomen)

ulcerated sore throat

(Source: Felter and Lloyd, 1898)

Meyer's formula was skillfully crafted, from an herbalist's point of view, for the conditions he lists. Wormwood *(Artemisia absinthum)* was commonly used as a cooling bitter tonic in Meyer's time, and a related species is used in China today to lower fever in malaria. Hops *(Humulus lupulus)* was also used as a bitter tonic to lower fevers, and especially to produce relaxation. It was also used externally on ulcers and tumors (Felter and Lloyd, 1898). This formula, combining echinacea with bitter herbs, is not unlike contemporary commercial formulas that combine echinacea with the very bitter goldenseal, although the modern rationale is different. It is also an excellent formula for external applications. I will discuss bitter tonics in more detail in Chapter 12.

Most prominent among Meyer's claims to King and Lloyd was the assertion that his remedy could cure rattlesnake bite. He provided the histories of 613 cases of rattlesnake bite in men and animals, all supposedly successfully treated. The Eclectic Ellingwood relates an experiment that Meyer performed on himself:

> *With the courage of his convictions upon him, he injected the venom of the crotalus [rattlesnake] into the first finger of his left hand; the swelling was rapid and in six hours was up to the elbow. At this time he took a dose of the remedy, bathed the part thoroughly, and laid down to pleasant dreams. On awakening in four hours, the pain and swelling were gone.*
>
> (Ellingwood, 1919)

Meyer even offered to send a rattlesnake to Dr. King so that he could perform experiments in treating snake-bitten animals with his medication. When King declined the offer, Meyer offered to come to Cincinnati himself and let himself be bitten by the snake. This offer was also declined, but it must have gotten the attention of Dr. King, who subsequently performed experiments with echinacea that eventually supported most of Meyer's claims.

Box 2.2 lists conditions for which King and several of his contemporary Eclectics found echinacea useful. King even experimented with echinacea on his wife, who had suffered from a "virulent cancer" for some years. King had tried to relieve her pain with every remedy at his disposal, but without great success. The echinacea apparently greatly relieved her pain until she eventually died (Lloyd, 1924). Fifteen years later, Eclectic cancer specialist Eli Jones would conclude, after performing his own experiments, that echinacea does not cure cancer, but does help relieve pain in terminal cases.

The Eclectics were naturally suspicious of Meyer's original claims, because they seemed so excessive. Many "patent medicines" of dubious nature were sold at that time with claims of miraculous cures. Felter later commented on Meyer's wide-ranging claims:

Subsequent use of the drug has in a measure substantiated the seeming incredulous claims of its introducer, for it will be observed that most of these conditions were such as might be due to blood deprivation, or to noxious introductions from without the body—the very field in which echinacea is known to display its power.

(Felter and Lloyd, 1898)

BOX 2.2
CONDITIONS FOR WHICH THE ECLECTICS SUCCESSFULLY USED ECHINACEA

blood poisoning

cerebral meningitis

cholera

chronic leg ulcers

diarrhea

dog bites

dysentery

eczema

gonorrhea

gastritis (chronic)

hemorrhoids

obstinate catarrh
[mucous]

pain due to swelling

poison ivy

psoriasis

rheumatism

stings of wasps and
bees with extensive
swelling

syphilis

ulcers

uterine infections

vaginal infection
with ulceration

The Eclectics accepted echinacea at first on King's authority, and eventually proved its worth in their own experience. Thus King, who had first mentioned echinacea to fellow professionals in his 1852 *Dispensatory*, and who died in 1893, made this tremendous final contribution to humanity in the sunset of his life. I will cover the Eclectic uses of echinacea in great detail in Chapter 3.

THE HOMEOPATHS

Within a decade of its introduction to Eclectic medicine by Dr. King, homeopaths were using *E. angustifolia* in the U.S., England, and Germany, and by the turn of the century its use became even more widespread. It first appeared formally in homeopathic literature in Clarke's *Practical Dictionary* (Clarke, 1902), wherein Clarke described his own clinical successes with the tincture. Clarke mentioned *E. purpurea* as an aside, but named no therapeutic uses. By 1906, *E. angustifolia* appeared in German homeopathic literature, and by the 1930s it was widely used by German physicians (Madaus, 1938). The homeopaths used it most often in the tincture form in doses of from five to forty drops. Box 2.3 shows the homeopathic uses of echinacea. At least seventy-five homeopathic products containing echinacea are sold in Germany today (Bauer and Wagner, 1990).

EUROPEAN USE

By the 1930s, *Echinacea angustifolia* was widely used in Europe, and large quantities were imported each year from the U.S. According to Foster, almost the entire export crop was bought by the French in 1937, creating a shortage for German firms. Dr. Gerhard Madaus, of the firm Madaus and Co., traveled to the U.S. that year to obtain seeds so that his company could grow its own supply (Foster, 1991). He bought what he thought were seeds of *E. angustifolia*, but when he planted them *E. purpurea* came up in the garden.

BOX 2.3

CONDITIONS TREATED WITH ECHINACEA
BY HOMEOPATHS

cancer (to ease pain
in final stages)

cold sores

crushing injuries

hemorrhoids
(external use)

lymphatic
inflammation

tooth abscesses

wounds (for healing
and disinfection)

(Source: Murphy, 1995)

This historical accident had huge implications for the world-wide use of echinacea. Upon experimentation, Madaus found that *E. purpurea* had medicinal properties similar to those of *E. angustifolia*. The Madaus company developed an ointment and liquid form for external use, an extract for internal use, and several forms for injection.

Unlike the previous echinacea products, Madaus used the flowering tops of *E. purpurea* — both leaves and flowers instead of the roots. His products were made from the juice of the flowering tops, stabilized with a small amount of alcohol (twenty-two percent). No record exists in the scientific literature on echinacea to show that he did comparison trials of the *E. purpurea* root and flowering tops before producing these items. I speculate that Madaus came upon this form in two ways. First, the German homeopaths made their *E. angustifolia* preparations from the whole flowering plant — root and tops—whereas the Eclectics had used only the root. Perhaps this was Madaus' inspiration to investigate the tops. Second, Madaus' chief concern was consistent supply. The echinacea plant is perennial, so he could harvest the tops without having to plant a new crop each year. New tops would grow each year from the same roots. If he had used the root, he would have had to wait two years to harvest each replanted crop. Thus, his decision to use the tops may have been as much a practical industrial one as a medicinal one.

Most of the subsequent echinacea research has been into the Madaus products. As a result, a huge disparity has developed between the products investigated by science and those used most often clinically. The German commission that regulates herbal products issued a monograph in 1990, based on the extensive research into the Madaus products, permitting the sale of flowering tops of *E. purpurea*. Due to lack of research, however, it denied monographs for the roots of *E. purpurea* or *E. angustifolia*, the latter being the form which the Eclectics used with such clinical success for almost fifty years. In Chapters 5 and 6, I will review the scientific research into echinacea, including the clinical reports of German physicians over the last fifty years.

CONCLUSION

Echinacea was introduced into medical practice by the Eclectics through more than forty years of practice and experimentation. In the next chapter, I will describe the Eclectic use in great detail, including the diseases treated and the forms and dosages used. In my opinion, the North American consumer today will find more practical information in the Eclectic uses than in the more abstract scientific research.

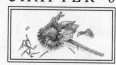

CHAPTER 3

THE ECLECTIC
USE OF
ECHINACEA

That a simple drug should possess such varied and remarkable therapeutic forces and not be a poison itself is an enigma still to be solved. And one that must come as a novelty to those whose therapy is that of heroic medicines only.

H.W. Felter

I briefly described the Eclectic school of medicine in the last chapter. Here I'll tell its story in more detail and explain how these physicians used echinacea to treat a wide range of both mild and life-threatening illnesses. In the next chapters, I'll describe scientific research into echinacea, but I would encourage you to pay more attention to this chapter; here you can learn how actual physicians used the same forms of echinacea that you can buy in any health-food store today—information as relevant to you as it was to them.

The history of Eclectic medicine is one of the best-kept secrets of American history. These physicians were an important presence in American medicine from 1830 to 1930, and we owe our knowledge of echinacea and its remarkable properties to them. Our contemporary medical histories are the product of the Regular school of medicine, which evolved into our current conventional medicine, and which had great disregard for the Eclectics. The Regulars swept the Eclectic school into oblivion in the first decades of this century by using political clout to deny accreditation to their schools and licensing to their practitioners.

In the process, the Eclectics were also swept from the medical history books. To get their story, you have to read their own literature and medical texts. On my bookshelf, within easy reach, I keep five of their medical texts totaling almost five thousand pages. In them is contained the most detailed clinical record of the medical-level use of Western herbs in the world. These doctors have had a profound influence, if not on conventional medicine, at least on contemporary naturopathic and homeopathic medicine, European conventional medicine, and on all schools of modern herbalism.

In 1830, the Regular school of medicine was dominated by dogmatism: "My theories are correct, clinical facts be damned." They used such drastic and injurious techniques as bloodletting, violent purgatives, and poisonous minerals such as mercury—and little else. These treatments are as likely to kill some patients as the diseases they suffer from. George Washington died at the hands of one of these doctors who literally bled him to death trying to cure a case of laryngitis.

A number of the Regular school members began to rebel against the use of such methods in the first decades of the nineteenth century. By the late 1820s, they were organized into the Reformed Medical Society by Dr. Wooster

Beach and several associates. By 1845, the Reformed school was called the Eclectic school. While maintaining their level of knowledge of basic medical sciences, these medical rebels turned to gentler, less drastic clinical methods, especially the use of herbs instead of mineral and chemical medicines. In 1830, they were rebels without anything to call their own, but over the next thirty years they assimilated methods and medicines from the unlicensed herbal practitioners of their day.

Around 1830, the botanist-physician Constantine Rafinesque, described in Chapter 2, adopted the word "Eclectic" to describe this practice of assimilating anything useful they could find in any school of medicine. This principle of assimilation and non-dogmatism characterized the Eclectics throughout their history, and they became the repository for much of what was clinically useful in the field of medical herbalism in North America during that period. Their later texts, written between 1910 and 1925, became something like Noah's Ark, carrying this assimilated and refined herbal knowledge across the flood of conventional medicine to the 1970s, when alternative schools began to make a resurgence. I was introduced to these texts at the National College of Naturopathic Medicine in Portland, Oregon, in the 1980s, and have studied them continuously ever since. These books are still available from Eclectic Medical Publications in Portland, or from the American Botanical Council in Austin, Texas (see Appendix 3).

The history of echinacea in medical practice is intimately interwoven with the history of the Eclectics. Rafinesque was the first to describe the uses of echinacea in a medical text (Rafinesque, 1830). The Eclectic professor John King described it further in the first Eclectic materia medica (King, 1852). And eventually it was King, thirty-five

years later, who substantiated Dr. Meyer's claims for echinacea, and, on the strength of his reputation, introduced it to
the profession.

Over the next forty years, the Eclectics experimented
extensively with echinacea, refining their preparations of it
and establishing the indications for its use. They even performed the first formal clinical experiments with it. By 1920,
echinacea was the top-selling medicine sold by the Lloyd
Brothers Pharmaceutical Company of Cincinnati, outselling
the next three remedies on the list put together. Box 3.1
shows a brief summary of its introduction to the world of
medicine. By 1939, when the last of the Eclectic medical
schools graduated its last class, echinacea had all but fallen
from use in North America by licensed physicians, except for
the few surviving Eclectics and members of the Naturopathic school of medicine.

THE ECLECTIC CLINICAL GIANTS

Before I describe how the Eclectics used echinacea, let me
introduce you to the three great physicians whose texts I've
used as sources. You will see that, using these authors as au-
thorities, I am not describing the properties of some fad
herb; I am describing one of the favorite remedies of three
masters of clinical medicine.

Dr. Harvey Wickes Felter

Felter was one of the great clinicians and educators of
the Eclectic medical movement. He started out practicing as
a Regular M.D. in New England, but after some disillusion-
ment he moved to Cincinnati, Ohio—the most important

BOX 3.1

TEXT FROM A 1921 ADVERTISEMENT FOR ECHINACEA BY THE LLOYD BROTHERS PHARMACEUTICAL COMPANY

Originally employed by the Indians and Pioneers

1885   Announced by the itinerant physician Dr. Meyer

1887   Introduced to the profession by Dr. John King

1890   A tincture was prepared for the use of investigating physicians, but not advertised

1894   Label prepared by Dr. Felter giving therapeutic uses

1899   First advertisement in a medical journal

1917   First historically descriptive pamphlet

1920   Heads the list of plant preparations, Lloyd Brothers laboratory

(Source: Bauer and Wagner, 1990)

center of Eclecticism in the U.S. He graduated at the top of his class from the Eclectic Medical Institute in 1888. He then became first an instructor, then Professor of Surgical Anatomy at the school. Eventually he became President of the National Eclectic Medical Association, and Professor of Materia Medica and Therapeutics and of the History of Medicine at the Eclectic Medical College in Cincinnati. In 1898 he co-authored, with pharmacist John Uri Lloyd, the classic *King's American Dispensatory*. This two-thousand-plus page book is the most thorough description of the medicinal use of North American plants in existence, and is available in reprint form today.

In 1922, Felter published *The Eclectic Materia Medica, Pharmacology, and Therapeutics*, a smaller book in which he attempted to collect the body of Eclectic experience with herbal medicines while eliminating the exaggerations and unrestrained enthusiasm to which medical writing of the day was prone. He was successful at his task of creating a credible, accurate, and useful materia medica; the text is still used in naturopathic medical colleges in the U.S. Coming late in the history of the Eclectics, this volume was a refinement of thirty-five years of clinical practice and observation.

Dr. Finley Ellingwood

Finley Ellingwood, whose career paralleled that of Felter, was Professor of Chemistry at Bennett Medical College in Chicago from 1884 to 1898. He authored a number of medical texts, including *Ellingwood's Practice of Medicine* and *Ellingwood's Pregnancy and Labor*. He was also editor of *Ellingwood's Therapeutist*, and of the *Chicago Medical Times*. He also began publishing editions of his *American Materia Medica*,

Therapeutics, and Pharmacognosy in 1898. The final edition appeared in 1919, and reprints are still available. Thus his later editions, like Felter's work, are refinements based on several decades of experience in medical practice. He says of echinacea:

> *For twenty to twenty-five years, echinacea has been passing through the stages of critical experimentation under the observation of several thousand physicians, and its remarkable properties are receiving positive confirmation. . . . All who use it correctly fall quickly into line as enthusiasts in its praise.*

(Ellingwood, 1919)

Ellingwood's passion was to promote knowledge of the specific medicinal properties of American plant medicines among all branches of medicine. As a medical editor and professor, he came in contact with and corresponded with many physicians of all the schools. He suggests that the last edition of his materia medica contains, directly or indirectly, the observations of more than twenty-five thousand practicing physicians. He states:

> *I have been encouraged to undertake this work; indeed I have felt a conscientious impulsion to undertake it, from the almost universal praise, commendation, and congratulations received from the thoughtful, successful, practical men of every*

school of medicine. It would be practically impossible to declare which school has been the most generous in their patronage.

(Ellingwood, 1919)

Dr. Eli Jones

Eli Jones devoted his entire career to clinical work, rather than teaching in schools, and was the master clinician of the Eclectic school of medicine. He was such a remarkable physician that I would like to write an entire book about him, but I'll have to confine myself to a few paragraphs. Although he ended up an Eclectic, his career took him through four schools of medicine.

Jones began practice as a Regular physician. After about five years, he abandoned the methods of that school and used homeopathy exclusively. After another five years, he began to practice using almost exclusively the twelve "tissue salts"—homeopathic-like remedies that entered into American medicine in the 1880s. Seeking to learn one "therapeutic fact" a day, Jones mastered each of the above disciplines until he could treat the whole range of human illness with each. Finally, he became an Eclectic and used their herbal remedies almost exclusively for a time. Only then did he consider himself a mature physician.

By this time, Jones had come into great demand as a teacher and held post-graduate courses for physicians of all schools in his office. He had also earned a reputation as a cancer specialist—the first such specialist in American history—and took referrals from all schools. His two great works are *Definite Medication: Containing Therapeutic Facts*

Gleaned from Forty Years Practice and *Cancer: Its Causes, Symptoms and Treatment,* both of which, unfortunately, are out of print. The strength of Jones' books is in their practical, rather than theoretical, content. He states:

> *In all my writings, I have been very careful about the statements that I made concerning a remedy, unless it has been tested by myself, not upon rats, mice, and rabbits, but at the bedside of the sick.*
>
> (Jones, 1911a)

THE GENERAL INDICATION FOR ECHINACEA: "BAD BLOOD"

The Eclectics viewed "bad blood" as the most important underlying condition that called for echinacea, and they called echinacea a "blood purifier." These older medical terms have as much relevance today as they did then, although they have fallen from use. Contemporary conventional physicians don't treat "bad blood," but wait for that physiological state to manifest as a specific disease before providing treatment. Then they usually treat the symptoms without addressing the underlying cause.

Millions of Americans are walking around today with bad blood, suffering from any number of uncomfortable symptoms or recurring illnesses arising from it. The "blood" of bad blood is not really the blood at all, but the extracellular fluid that bathes the cells. The blood itself only comprises about five percent of the fluids in the body, while the extracellular fluid makes up about twenty percent. This extracellular fluid accumulates the metabolic wastes of all the cells, the waste products of infection and inflammation, and the toxic byproducts of poor digestion. When an infection spreads, it spreads through this medium.

The extracellular fluid must be purified first by elements of the immune system called *phagocytes*. (I'll explain the immune system in detail in Chapter 4.) Whatever is left, including the dead phagocytes, is purified by the lymphatic system, which drains the dead toxic components through a series of lymph nodes, where the immune system eliminates them. When the load is too great for the phagocytes and the elements in the lymph nodes to handle, "bad blood" occurs. It is possible for an infection to spread to the actual blood; this condition, termed *septicemia*, is potentially fatal.

The Eclectics routinely treated and cured even septicemia with echinacea. Today we know echinacea as an "immune stimulant," and it should be clear that this is not incompatible with the eclectic term of "blood purifier," because the immune system has such a predominant role in purifying the "blood." In Box 3.2, I list some of the symptoms that can arise from bad blood. Bad blood may also arise from external poisonings, such as snake, scorpion, or insect bites.

THE ACTIONS OF ECHINACEA

Physicians and modern herbalists alike classify herbs by their actions, or the effects they produce in the body. Most herbs have multiple actions, and echinacea is no exception. Table 3.1 lists the actions of echinacea.

BOX 3.2
SOME MEDICAL SYMPTOMS THAT MAY ARISE FROM "BAD BLOOD"

abscesses	gangrene
boils	malignant tumors
chronic infection	mental disturbances
chronic inflammation	psoriasis
eczema	septicemia
emaciation	skin ulcers
fever	swollen glands
foul discharges	

Alterative Properties

The traditional herbal treatment for bad blood is *alterative* therapy, using alterative herbs. The term comes from the word "to alter," meaning to change the composition and quality of the extracellular fluid and blood. The Eclectics considered echinacea to be the Queen of the Alteratives, and Felter states: "If there is any meaning in the term *alterative*, it is expressed in the therapy of echinacea." Echinacea works

TABLE 3.1   THE PROPERTIES OF ECHINACEA

Alterative	Purifies the blood and lymph
Anesthetic	Relieves local pain
Anti-putrefactive	Combats the breakdown of tissues during infection
Antipyretic	Lowers fever
Antiseptic	Fights infection topically
Appetizer	Promotes the appetite
Deodorant	Reduces the foul smell of infection
Depurative	Promotes the removal of foul excretions
Diuretic	Promotes the flow of urine
Sialagogue	Promotes the flow of saliva
Stimulant	Increases circulation to local tissues
Tonic	Builds overall health

primarily on the immune system, but other alteratives might also act to stimulate the body's own purification processes, including liver, bowel, and kidney function. I will describe other alteratives in later chapters of the book.

Antipyretic Properties

The Eclectics observed that echinacea would lower fevers caused by bacterial infections. They used it routinely in such serious illnesses as typhoid and scarlet fever. Ellingwood describes this effect in several infections following childbirth:

In several cases reported of septic womb ... the temperature has declined from one-half to two degrees within a few hours after its use was begun, and has not increased until the agent was discontinued. It has then increased toward the previous high point until the remedy was again taken, when a decline was soon apparent. It does not produce abrupt drops in temperature ... but it effects an almost immediate stop in germ development, and a steady restoration from its pernicious influence.

(Ellingwood, 1919)

Antiseptic Properties

Antiseptics prevent infection by inhibiting the growth and spread of bacteria. The Eclectics applied echinacea topically on wounds to prevent infection before it set in. This is identical to an original Native American use of the plant. They would also apply it to already infected wounds, skin ulcers, and any sort of skin infection. Felter states:

The greater the tendency to lifelessness and dissolution of the tissues and the more pronounced the fetid discharges, the more applicable is echinacea.

(Felter, 1922)

The Eclectics used echinacea as a disinfectant during surgery, to dress the surgical incision to prevent infection.

They also used it internally during surgery, directly on internal organs where infectious abscesses or tumors were removed, or in the abdominal cavity if septic contents had been discharged there during the operation (Felter, 1898, 1922).

Sialagogue Properties

One of the first things you notice after taking a dose of *Echinacea angustifolia* is tingling in the mouth. Shortly thereafter, your saliva starts to flow more profusely—a *sialagogue* effect. Ellingwood held that echinacea has a similar effect on the internal glands—the digestive secretions—and that the general nutrition is improved by this influence.

Stimulant Properties

When traditional herbalists speak of a *stimulant*, they are not talking about your morning cup of coffee. An herbal stimulant improves the blood circulation, especially to the capillaries—the tiniest vessels that supply blood to the cells. We know today that echinacea stimulates the immune system at the level of the white blood cells. But it also increases the flow of blood to the tissues, an action that modern scientists have overlooked. Thus it not only possesses weapons against infection, it has its own stimulating delivery system to get them where they are needed. Felter says of echinacea:

> *As a stimulant to the capillary circulation, no remedy is comparable with it, and it endows the vessels with a recuperative power or formative force, so as to*

enable them to successfully resist local inflammatory
processes due to debility and blood deprivation.

(Felter and Lloyd, 1898)

Ellingwood cites as evidence of this stimulant power
the fact that "sallow, pallid, and dingy" conditions of the skin
and the face quickly disappear, and the "rosy hue of health
becomes apparent." The pink look of the skin is due to the
increased circulation of blood there.

ECHINACEA NOT A CURE-ALL

Despite these potent medicinal effects, the Eclectics warned
that echinacea is not a cure-all, although it is a valuable adjunct to the primary remedies. Says Felter (1922):

So important is its antiseptic action that we are in-
clined to rely largely on it as an auxiliary remedy in
the more serious varieties of disease —even those with
a decided malignancy, such as diphtheria, smallpox,
scarlet fever, typhoid fever and typhoid pneumonia,
cerebrospinal meningitis, la grippe, uraemia, and the
surgical, serpent, and insect infections.

Thus the eclectics used echinacea *along with* other
remedies in more serious conditions. Notice that *la grippe* is
mentioned. This is an older name for the flu. In Chapter 17, I
will describe the advisability of using other herbs, either
alone or in combination with echinacea, for the flu.

DOSAGE

The Eclectics used a wide dose range for echinacea, but the most common was between ten and twenty drops every two or three hours. This is about one-half to a full dropper from a tincture bottle. Practitioners today are inclined to give larger doses less frequently, such as thirty to sixty drops three or four times a day. This Eclectic dose frequency was so universal among the writers that we would do well to follow their wisdom in the matter. It seems, from their experience, that *frequency* is more important than a high dose—that it is more important to keep the immune system constantly stimulated during an illness than to give massive doses with less frequency. Most Americans, and indeed most herbalists today, accustomed to high doses of powerful pharmaceutical drugs, do not have faith in such lower doses. Consider the following two cases as evidence of their potency.

Case One: Septic Abortion

Extreme septic absorption after a badly conducted abortion caused acute nephritis [kidney infection] and suppression of the urine. Uraemia [excess of normal urinary wastes in the blood], with delirium and mild convulsions. Twenty drops of the fluid extract of echinacea were given every two hours continuously. Extreme heat was applied over the kidneys, and a single dose of an antispasmodic (for the convulsions) was given, the echinacea alone being continued. The fever dropped in two days, the mind

cleared, the urinary secretion was restored, and the
patient made a rapid and uninterrupted recovery.

(Ellingwood, 1919)

Case Two: Vaccine Poisoning

Earlier in this century, it was not unusual for individuals to become quite ill after receiving vaccinations. Here is one such case treated with echinacea.

A gentleman, aged about forty-five years, in appar-
ently good health, was vaccinated, and as the result
of supposed impure vaccine a most unusual train of
the symptoms supervened. His vitality began to
wane, and he became so weak that he could not sit up.
His hair came out, and a skin disease pronounced by
experts to be psoriasis appeared upon his extremities
first, and afterward upon his body. In the writer's
opinion, the condition had but little resemblance to
psoriasis. It seemed more like an acute development
of leprosy than any other known conditions. This ad-
vanced rapidly, his nails began to fall off, he lost
flesh, and an iritis of the left eye developed and ulcer-
ation of the cornea in the right set in. After some
conventional medications, the hair loss stopped, but
no other favorable results were obtained. The condi-
tion progressed rapidly toward an apparently fatal

termination, At this juncture, Dr. Martin asked the writer to see the case with him. It looked as if there was no possible salvation for the patient, but as a last resort, the writer suggested echinacea, twenty drops every two hours. With this treatment, in from four to six weeks, the patient regained his normal weight of more than 150 pounds and enjoyed afterward as good health as ever in his life.

(Ellingwood, 1919)

Smaller and Larger Doses

Eli Jones often used doses smaller than Ellingwood used on the vaccine-poisoned patient, for equally serious conditions. His usual dose was five to ten drops every two or three hours, although he would occasionally use doses as high as sixty drops.

Felter stated in 1898 that larger doses, even sixty drops, might be employed, but said that small doses frequently repeated are most effective. He also advocated massive doses in certain life-threatening conditions.

I am convinced that success in certain cases depends upon the fact that the patient must have at times a sufficiently large quantity of this remedy in order to produce full antitoxic effects on the virulent infections. I would therefore emphasize the statements which I have previously made that it is perfectly safe

to give echinacea in massive doses—from two drams
[about one-eighth ounce] to half an ounce every two
or three hours, for a time at least, when the system is
overwhelmed with these toxins. This applies to
tetanus, anthrax, actinomycosis, pyemia, diph-
theria, hydrophobia, and meningitis.

(Felter, 1898)

CANCER

The Eclectics used echinacea for cancer, but never considered it a cure for that disease. Professor King, who first introduced echinacea into medical practice, used the remedy
to treat his own wife, who had terminal cancer. He reported that it was the only thing that would ease her pain.
Twenty years later, cancer specialist Eli Jones, after treating
thousands of cancer patients, stated clearly that echinacea
was not a cure, but that it would indeed reduce pain in the
later stages.

POISONOUS BITES AND STINGS

We saw in the last chapter that echinacea earned its early
fame as a cure for rattlesnake bites. This use was extensively
verified by the Eclectics. Ellingwood cites a case of tarantula
bite in which echinacea "quickly eliminated" all trace of the
poison.

I had my own experience with echinacea and a scorpion bite. I was bitten on the arm one night while sitting in

the desert under a full moon near my hotel in Tempe, Arizona. At first I thought I had stuck myself on a cactus spine. Then, as the poison entered my system, I got a rash on my feet that started creeping up my legs. I thought that perhaps I had brushed against some poisonous plant, not connecting the sting in my arm with the rash on my legs. I went inside and took a hot shower to wash off whatever "poison" was on my skin, and went to bed. I noticed that my pulse was racing—about one hundred beats per minute, up from a normal of around seventy. I thought that this racing pulse might be due to the stress of travel and the conference I was attending.

When I awoke in the morning my pulse was still at one hundred, and I realized that something was wrong. The sting on my arm had gotten ugly; it looked as if the skin around it was already dead. I immediately started taking echinacea—a teaspoonful every two hours—and a homeopathic remedy for stings. I also drank large amounts of water to wash the poison out of my system. In the afternoon I took a nap. When I awoke I was fine, just like Dr. Meyer when he awoke from his nap after injecting rattlesnake venom and taking echinacea. I now have only a scar from the initial sting to show for it. Later I learned that my symptoms matched those of the bite of the scorpion *Centruroides exilicauda,* one of the few seriously poisonous scorpions in North America.

FORMS OF ECHINACEA APPLICATION

The Eclectics used echinacea in a variety of applications, several of which North American herbalists and physicians seem to have forgotten completely. The most important of these is the external application. The Native Americans had used echinacea both internally and externally, and we saw in Chapter 2 that Dr. Meyer, when treating his own self-induced snakebite, took echinacea internally and also bathed his swollen arm with it. The eclectics used diluted echinacea tincture as a wash, not only for infected wounds, but for conditions such as severe poison ivy, bee stings, spider bites, eczema, and psoriasis. The dilution was from one to sixty percent, and the most common was about one part echinacea tincture to six parts water. The stronger applications were reserved for poisonous bites and stings or severe infections. A saturated compress would be applied every two hours or, if necessary, more often. One contemporary topical antiseptic product, Absorbine Junior contains echinacea along with pot marigold *(Calendula officinalis)*, wormwood *(Artemisia absinthum)*, and menthol (Awang, 1991). This may be a surviving "patent medicine" with a new package.

THE LLOYD BROTHERS PHARMACY PRODUCTS

Eclectic pharmacist John Uri Lloyd was the main supplier of medicines to the Eclectic profession. His most important products, called "specific medicines," were not simple alcohol tinctures such as we use today. Through extensive experimentation, he made sophisticated extractions which concentrated certain constituents and removed others. His company sold hundreds of such extracts. None of his formulas survive, unfortunately, which is a great loss for North American herbalists. Lloyd Brothers sold four echinacea products:

TABLE 3.2   SOME ECLECTIC METHODS OF
APPLYING ECHINACEA

Compress	Diluted tincture, for wounds, skin afflictions, poison ivy, or boils.
Douche	Diluted tincture, for vaginal and uterine infections.
Enema	Diluted tincture, for hemorrhoids or anal infections.
Fluid extract	One part plant material to one part solvent for internal use.
Spray	Diluted tincture for nasal, sinus, and throat infections.
Tincture	One part echinacea to five parts 80-percent alcohol solution for internal use.

- Specific Echinacea, a proprietary concentrated extract of echinacea
- Echafolta, a clear echinacea liquid extract with the coloring matter removed, for use in surgery or in open wounds
- Iodized Echafolta, which included iodine for its antiseptic properties
- Echafolta Cream, for external applications

CONCLUSION

As the sun of the Eclectic profession was setting in the 1930s, echinacea's sun was rising in Germany. By the end of that decade, the Madaus pharmaceutical company began growing and marketing echinacea products, and they have remained popular ever since, both among physicians and consumers in that country. The Germans eventually began scientific research into echinacea, and today account for most of the published research into the plant and its constituents. In Chapters 5 and 6, I'll review the scientific research into echinacea, but first, in the next chapter, I'll introduce you to the wonders of the immune system. You will need at least an overview of its components in order to understand the significance of the scientific research that follows.

CHAPTER 4

THE IMMUNE
SYSTEM

To understand how echinacea, goldenseal, and other immune-system-stimulating herbs work, you'll need a basic understanding of how the immune system operates. Immunology is still a young science—born in the late 1800s—with new discoveries occurring every year. An entire major branch of the immune system—cell-mediated immunity—was discovered in the 1940s. Only a few basic facts about the immune system were understood as recently as the 1970s. With the advent of the AIDS epidemic, and with ongoing research into that disease and into cancer, the amount of knowledge has mushroomed dramatically. Most of what we now know of the fine details of immunology has been discovered in the last twenty years. Some of the immunology I learned at medical school in 1986 is now obsolete, only ten years later. The knowledge of the interactions of herbs with this system is even newer than the science itself, although many of the immune-system-stimulating herbs have been traditionally used as "blood purifiers" and "tonics." In this chapter, I'll give a general overview of the immune system that I hope won't be obsolete while the book is still in print.

SELF AND OTHER

The human body is a collection of about seventy-five billion cells, all coordinated and interconnected. If each cell were the size of a child's marble, and they were packed together on a flat surface, they would make a band wider than a football field that would stretch all the way around the equator of the earth. These billions of cells rest in a matrix of connective tissue where they are constantly bathed by the extracellular fluids, which make up about a fifth of the liquid content of the body. Blood circulation and other physiological mechanisms work to keep the consistency of this extracellular fluid constant. The blood itself contains only 5 percent of the fluids in the body, and is actually extracellular fluid "in transit," circulating both nutrients and wastes in order to maintain the steady state of the extracellular fluid.

Like the oceans of the earth, the extracellular fluid has essentially the same composition throughout the body. In fact, it has a salty mineral content very similar to that of the oceans, and is literally the "inner sea" of the body that nourishes each of the cells. This mass of cells nourished by its inner sea is wrapped in skin, supported by bones, and equipped with organs for sensing, moving about, acquiring nutrition, eliminating wastes, and maintaining consciousness; it is invigorated by the vital force of the body. With the help of another organism, it can even make a copy resembling itself.

A miracle of creation is the ability of this organism to maintain its distinct identity—its unique "self"—while moving about in a vast biological environment, assimilating food and breathing air laden with microscopic organisms, coexisting with hundreds of millions of bacteria and other organisms that live in its intestines and on its skin, removing the debris of its own dead cells (more than 300,000,000 die each day) and policing and destroying any of its cells that tend to stray and become life-threatening, cancerous renegades. Separated from both the outer environment and the toxic sewer of the digestive tract by only a single layer of cells, our organism still manages to maintain its uniqueness. The mechanisms of the body that maintain this "selfness" in the face of constant assault by the environment may collectively be called the immune system.

The three levels of the immune system for maintaining the biological "self" are: barriers, non-specific defenses, and specific defenses. The barriers are like the walls of your house, the non-specific defenses are like the burglar alarm and your guard dogs, and the specific defenses are like well-aimed firearms in the hands of a homeowner that carefully determines whether an intruder is friend or foe. In the body, the three levels are profoundly interconnected, and indeed do not exist entirely independently of each other. The herbs I discuss in this book work at these various levels, and echinacea works at all three.

BARRIERS

The barrier defenses present physical obstacles to invasion by foreign cells or particles. The skin is composed of tightly packed cells with an intercellular cement between then. The mucous membranes are specialized "skin" that can secrete sticky fluids to trap and wash away invaders. Mucus-covered

nasal hairs also trap dust particles and bacteria. Other secretions wash away invaders or kill them: saliva, stomach acid,
digestive juices, the oily secretions of the skin, tears, urine,
and the secretions of the vagina and the prostate gland. Some
of these, including stomach acid, urine, and the secretions
of the reproductive organs, contain microorganism-killing
acids. Others, including mucus, the oily secretions of the
skin, tears, and saliva, contain antibiotic substances.

The Hyaluronic Acid/
Hyaluronidase System

One of the key barrier defenses is the hyaluronic acid
system in the connective tissue of the body. Starting at the
surface of your skin, and present in every part of your body,
a mucus-like connective tissue holds the cells of your body in
place. It prevents particles, bacteria, viruses, and other invaders from moving freely within the body. This tissue is saturated with the extracellular fluid of the "inner sea"
described above, and is the medium through which fluids
seep back and forth between the capillaries of your blood
vessels and the cells themselves, or drain into your lymph
vessels, a network of vessels resembling the veins that trans-
port extracellular fluid and wastes back toward the heart. The
fluid in the tissues is neither liquid nor solid, but in an inter-
mediate state something like jelly. This gel is part of the
"glue" that holds the body together. If the fluid in the connective tissue became watery, much of the material between
your skin and your bones would flow down and collect between your knees and ankles within a few minutes.

The stickiness of the fluid is produced by a balance between a thick hyaluronic acid secreted by connective tissue

cells, and hyaluronidase, which thins that secretion. If there is more hyaluronic acid or less hyaluronidase, the gel becomes thicker. We will see in Chapter 6 that some forms of echinacea thicken this intercellular "jelly," frustrating the passage of bacteria or viruses through the tissues; it also inactivates substances in some bacteria that allows them to "melt" the intercellular gel.

Non-Specific Defenses

The non-specific defenses are like the burglar alarm or the guard dogs in your house. Your dogs will bark at anyone they do not recognize, and, if necessary, bite them in the leg. This is non-specific, because they don't care who it is. They are not trained to attack one specific person. And their barking alerts the owner (the specific defense system). Similarly, if someone comes into your house who does not know the deactivation code for the burglar alarm, it will go off to waken the owner and summon the police, who will then identify the specific intruder and take appropriate action. Table 4.1 shows the elements of the non-specific defenses of the body.

Phagocytes

The most important of the non-specific defenses are the *phagocytes*. These include circulating white blood cells called *neutrophils* and *monocytes*, but especially cells called macrophages. All these cells have amoeba-like motion, and can slip through the blood vessel walls into the tissues to "eat" invaders there in a process called phagocytosis.

TABLE 4.1   NON-SPECIFIC CELLULAR AND
CHEMICAL DEFENSES OF THE
IMMUNE SYSTEM

Phagocytes	Engulf and destroy invading pathogens that breach the barrier defenses, and trigger the response of some of the specific immune system defenses
Natural killer cells (T-killer cells, cytotoxic T-cells)	Attack virally infected cells, cancerous cells, and foreign cells such as are found in organ transplants
Inflammatory response	Prevents the spread of invading organisms, removes pathogens and dead cells, attracts phagocytes and members of the specific immune system defense to the area, and promotes tissue repair
Fever response	Triggered by secretions of the phagocytes; promotes the rapid multiplication of immune system cells and enhances tissue repair
Antimicrobial chemicals	Freely circulating chemicals called the properidin-complement system enhance immune system and inflammatory responses and can also directly destroy invaders.

Macrophage means "big eater." The macrophages are fewer in number than the neutrophils and monocytes, but they can eat many more bacteria or other antigens—up to 100 each. They can even eat other blood cells whole—the cellular equivalent of a boa constrictor swallowing a donkey. Macrophages occur not only in the blood, but hundreds of millions of them line the lungs, liver, lymph nodes, spleen, and bone marrow. They are also spread throughout the connective tissue in the body.

Macrophages fit the analogy of guard dogs well, except that they eat intruders whole instead of just biting them. They then send chemical signals out to other parts of the immune system and stick parts of the eaten invader out of the surface of their membranes. These are recognized by the *T-helper cells* of the specific immune system, which I will describe below. The "handshake" between a macrophage that has eaten an invader and the T-cell that is sensitive to that invader is the most important event in the immune response, and stimulates all levels of the immune system. We'll see in Chapter 6 that echinacea increases the number and stimulates the activity of all the phagocytes.

Natural Killer Cells

Natural killer cells, also called *cytotoxic T-cells* are like the special-forces troops of non-specific immunity. They don't engulf the invaders like the phagocytes do, but they attach to the invaders and secrete poisons into them that kill them. Unlike a phagocyte, a natural killer cell can attack many invaders, one after another. They are indispensable in the body's fight against cancer cells and virally infected cells, which they kill on sight, rather than waiting for a larger immune system response to begin. They also attack foreign cells such as those found in organ transplants. Thus, a lifetime prescription of immunosuppressive drugs is necessary to suppress these T-cells after an organ transplant.

Inflammation

Inflammation, which can be triggered by injury or an immune system response, is characterized by symptoms of swelling, redness, and pain. It underlies dozens of disease conditions, depending on the tissue affected and the severity of the inflammation. Although uncomfortable, inflammation is a healthy process that is essential to immunity; Box 4.1 lists its benefits. The use of drugs to suppress inflammation makes an underlying condition worse by turning off what is by nature a healing reaction, especially if the drugs are used chronically. We will see in Chapter 6 that echinacea is appropriate for short-term use as an anti-inflammatory in acute inflammation such as bee stings or sunburn.

Fever

Fever is a healthy physiological reaction and is essential for the optimal operation of the immune system. Fever may be triggered by the presence of various chemicals in the blood, including those secreted by macrophages after they have eaten invaders. Heightened body metabolism causes the elevated fever as the body goes into overdrive, cranking up the system to produce and circulate more antibodies and white blood cells, to eliminate wastes and to repair tissues. Also during fever, large amounts of iron and zinc—favorite foods of invading bacteria—are pulled out of the blood and stored in the liver and spleen.

A normal, healthy fever is around 102 degrees Fahrenheit, and temperatures below 104 degrees for a few days generally present no health hazard. The practice of habitually suppressing normal fevers with aspirin can only harm the body in the long run. A healthier practice is to fast from foods during fever, drink plenty of liquids, and make yourself comfortable in bed. Although echinacea may lower

---

BOX 4.1

THE BENEFITS OF INFLAMMATION

- prevents the spread of microorganisms or other irritants

- increases the circulation of immune cells to the area to fight intruders

- promotes the removal of dead cells and bacteria

- promotes local healing

---

fever, it is not as suppressive as aspirin and other pharmaceutical drugs.

Antimicrobial Chemicals

A set of chemicals that circulates in the blood and extracellular fluid is known collectively as the *complement system*. These chemicals may kill bacteria or other cells directly, initiate inflammation, or assist immune system operations in other ways. Another chemical, called *interferon,* is secreted by virally infected cells and helps to protect neighboring cells from infection. Echinacea injections have been shown to increase the effect of both these chemical systems.

SPECIFIC DEFENSES

If the macrophages are like guard dogs that will bark at and eat any intruder they do not recognize, the specific immune system is like a police SWAT team that will shoot only known criminals. To be more precise, each member of the "SWAT team" can shoot only one particular criminal type. They can and do, however, call in as many cloned copies of themselves for reinforcement as are necessary to defeat that particular type of criminal. Table 4.2 shows the elements of the specific immune system. Three qualities that make this system unique are:

1. Specificity: This system reacts against specific substances, preprogrammed by the body's genetic makeup.
2. Systemic action: Unlike the non-specific defenses, which act only at the site of infection, the specific defense system activates immunity to the invading organism throughout the entire body.
3. Memory: The specific defenses "remember" an invading antigen and mount an even more massive attack if they see that antigen again.

Antigens

The trigger for the specific immune system is an *antigen* — any particle of matter that the immune system cells recognize as foreign. Antigens are often groups of proteins in the cell walls of bacteria, viruses, or other organisms — protein sequences not found in the human body. Most antigens are large complex molecules rather than actual microorganisms.

Humoral Immunity and Antibodies

Humoral immunity has nothing to do with the immune-system-stimulating power of comedy, but refers to immunity that is spread throughout the "humors," or circulating fluids, of the body. The essential element of humoral immunity is the *antibody*. These small proteins are targeted to specific antigens like a key to a specific lock. And once the antibody binds chemically to an antigen—the key is inserted in the lock—the antigen can be destroyed in several ways. The antibody may mask a dangerous portion of a bacterium, protecting the cells from infection. It may cause invading organisms or cells to clump together or to become soluble in the body fluids. It may mark the invading organism or molecule for destruction by the phagocytes or the complement system and sometimes also triggers inflammation.

B-Lymphocytes and Plasma Cells

Antibodies do not occur naturally in the body, but are manufactured by B-lymphocytes; these reside in lymphatic tissue, especially in the lymph nodes. The B-lymphocytes are genetically programmed to respond to certain antigens. After the maturation of the immune system, hundreds of millions of antigen-specific B-cells lie in wait for their particular targeted antigen. Once the encounter occurs, the B-cell begins to make millions of copies of itself, which in turn manufacture antibodies specific to the antigen that triggered the process.

Some of these copies, called *plasma cells*, are highly activated antibody factories. They produce antibodies at the unbelievable rate of two thousand antibody molecules per second—more than a billion antibodies a week from each plasma cell—and circulate them throughout the body. Other copies of the B-cells, called *memory-B-cells*, are circulated throughout the lymph tissues in the body, communicating the memory of the infection throughout the system. Subsequent invasions by that particular antigen don't stand a chance against such preparations. This is the process by which immunizations work. Bacteria or viruses which have been inactivated, but which still have the antigenic proteins in their cell walls, are injected to trigger the initial "infection." After that, the memory cells circulate throughout the lymphatics, and any future exposure to the antigens is met with a massive response.

Cell-Mediated Immunity and the T-Cells

The essential element of cell-mediated immunity is the T-helper cell, also called a T-4 cell. This is the cell that the HIV virus attacks. When its numbers decline sufficiently, the individual's immune system fails to protect the organism, and AIDS—Acquired Immuno-Deficiency Syndrome—is the result.

Unlike the B-cells, the T-helper cells cannot react to their preprogrammed antigens directly. The antigen must be handed to them by a phagocyte that has already eaten and partially digested an invader. The phagocyte first chemically attracts the T-cell, and then the antigen on the macrophage surface activates the T-cell. The helper cell then emits chemicals that cause the proliferation of other T-helper cells, plasma cells, and antibodies. It also attracts still more macrophages to the area and drives them into a "feeding

Table 4.2   The Specific Immune System

Antigens	Foreign particles that elicit an immune system response from B-cells or T-cells. The cells are pre-programmed to attack one specific antigen.

Humoral-mediated Immunity

Antibodies	Small proteins that circulate throughout the blood, extracellular fluid, and lymph, which are designed to attach to, neutralize, or destroy specific antigens.
B-lymphocytes (B-cells)	The lymphocyte cells responsible for initiating humoral immunity after recognizing the antigen they are programmed to attack.
Plasma cells	B-cells that have been transformed into antibody-producing factories, collectively producing billions of circulating antibodies to the antigen that initially triggered the B-cell.

Cell-mediated Immunity

T-helper cells	Respond only to antigens "handed" to them by phagocytes. The helper cell then emits chemicals that cause the proliferation of other T-helper cells, plasma cells, and antibodies. They attract still more phagocytes, drive them into a "feeding frenzy," and stimulate T-killer cells in the area.
T-killer cells	These are also listed under non-specific defenses because they can act without stimulation by specific antigens. They are also antigen-specific and are stimulated to activity by the T-helper cells.

frenzy," stimulating their powers of phagocytosis. The T-helper cells also stimulate T-killer cells in the area to activity.

Echinacea clearly stimulates phagocytosis, but it is not clear to what extent it stimulates or acts through the T-cells. As we will see in Chapter 6, several clinical trials have shown that it is especially effective in patients with low T-cell activity (Coeugniet and Kühnast, 1986; Schöneberger, 1992).

THEY CAME FROM PLANET X

The story of the human immune system response could make a prize-winning science fiction story. Invaders from Planet X (antigens) attack the mother planet (the body). They first penetrate the outer shield defenses of the planet (skin, mucous membranes, etc.). The civilization on the planet already knows about these invaders (genetic preprogramming) and have prepared specific defenses against them. Several of the invaders are captured, identified, and interrogated (phagocytes and B-cells).

The alarm is raised (phagocytes) and the planet is put on war footing (fever, inflammation). The army (T-helper cells) declares martial law and orders are then sent throughout the planet to set up weapons factories (plasma cells) that will manufacture weapons deadly to this particular invader. Within a few hours, billions of genetically engineered invader-specific weapons (antibodies) are being produced. These are rapidly circulated to every corner of the planet. The army institutes the draft (proliferation of more T-helper cells) and mobilizes local attacks by foot soldiers (attracts and activates phagocytes). It sends out special-forces troops (T-killer cells) to destroy any cities or towns of the planet in which the invader has established a foothold.

Afterward, mop-up operations (more phagocytes) remove the debris of battle, and clean-up crews (the last stages of inflammation and fever) rebuild and fortify any cities or towns that have been damaged. It sounds almost like the script to the movie *Independence Day,* except that the earthlings in this case would win the battle on the second or third day.

THE CIRCULATORY DYNAMICS OF THE IMMUNE SYSTEM

Most of the battle of the immune system occurs in the extracellular spaces, between the cells and the blood vessels. As I described earlier, this space is permeated by the "inner sea" of the extracellular fluid, which bathes, nourishes, and accepts wastes from the cells. The liquid portion of this inner sea, and anything dissolved in it, can leak back into the blood vessels to return to the heart through the veins. But large molecules and other materials can't get back into the blood vessels. They must be taken back to the general circulation system through the lymph. There are several kinds of materials from the extracellular fluid that must be washed from the extracellular spaces through the lymph vessels, to empty into the veins near the heart. These substances that are removed from the tissues by the lymphatic system include:

cancer cells
dead cells
digested fats
food particles compressed into the tonsils
invading bacteria and viruses
large molecules manufactured by the cells

Many of these materials would be poisonous—even deadly—to the body if they reached the general circulatory system. Bacteria and viruses may establish a foothold in

infected tissue and reproduce millions of copies of themselves each hour. A cancerous tumor may release from ten
million to one billion cancer cells into the tissues each day.
All of these must be killed by the immune system, or the infection or cancer will spread. Furthermore, approximately
three hundred million cells die each day in the body and
must be disposed of. Even the phagocytes of the immune
system eventually die after destroying invaders, and must be
removed.

Macrophages and other elements of the non-specific
immune system are scattered throughout the tissues, and
they may handle the dangerous elements in the extracellular
fluid. Anything that gets past the macrophages enters the
lymphatic vessels, so all along these vessels are a series of
lymph nodes which block and filter the materials. The lymph is
squeezed under pressure through the nodes, which are
packed with macrophages, B-cells, and T-helper cells. The
nodes are the main seat of the specific immune system in the
body. The B-cells, in fact, never leave the nodes, so in order
for a system-wide antibody response to occur, an antigen
must find its way into a node. The T-helper cells live in the
nodes, but also cycle freely through the lymphatics to the
blood, into the tissues, and then back to the nodes.

The anatomy of a lymph node is such that antigens
that flow into it are first exposed to the B-cells and
macrophages, then to T-helper cells, and finally to a mass of
more macrophages. As we saw above, the activation of the
T-cells by macrophages that have already processed an antigen is the key to triggering a full immune system response, so
the nodes are arranged to support this process. The T-cells in
the node then stimulate the mass of macrophages near the
exit into a feeding frenzy.

Some specialized lymphatic tissue acts as a surveillance system for the body. The back of the roof of the mouth, the back of the tongue, and the tonsils in the throat are packed with lymphatic tissue. They sample a little bit of whatever enters the body through the mouth, and, if necessary, set off a systemic immune system response to prepare for materials that may enter the blood through the digestive tract. Similar lymphatic tissue is located throughout the digestive tract and is concentrated in the appendix and in areas called Peyer's patches, near where the small intestine meets the large intestine. We will see in Chapter 6 that echinacea may trigger the body's immune system response through interaction with these lymphatics in the mouth, and that it may thus be important to taste your echinacea rather than consume it in capsules.

About two quarts of lymph move through the lymph vessels in the body each day—a small amount compared to the blood, which circulates thousands of times that volume. This flow of lymph is absolutely necessary for the healthy operation of the immune system. If the flow becomes stagnant, waste materials build up in the tissues, the body becomes overloaded with toxic materials, and the immune system is depressed. In Chapter 10, I will describe lifestyle factors that promote the healthy flow of lymph in the body. Healthy exercise, proper rest, and drinking plenty of liquids is essential for a healthy lymphatic system. In Chapter 19, I'll describe herbs that are traditionally considered to promote the flow of lymph.

CHAPTER 5

Echinacea Constituents

Dozens of constituents of echinacea have been isolated and investigated in the past hundred years, but there is no scientific consensus that any one of them is solely responsible for echinacea's medicinal effects. In fact, current opinion is that more than one constituent is responsible (Bauer and Wagner, 1991). The three main echinacea species have different chemical "fingerprints," and no comparative clinical trials have determined which, if any, has the strongest therapeutic effect in humans.

We can conveniently divide echinacea constituents into alcohol-soluble and water-soluble groups. Such a division will help you understand which constituents are present in herbal preparations such as tinctures, teas, or capsules; these may be made with varying amounts of alcohol or water, or with neither one. The alcohol-soluble constituents will be present in the whole plant or in a tincture. Some water-soluble constituents may also be present in a tincture, which is made from a mixture of water and alcohol, and some may not. Constituents that are only soluble in alcohol will not be present in a tea. The whole plant should theoretically contain all the substances, but if it has been dried, constituents soluble in either water or alcohol may degrade, and alcohol-soluble substances may evaporate.

ALCOHOL-SOLUBLE CONSTITUENTS

The alcohol-soluble constituents, as a group, are probably the most important of the immune-system-stimulating constituents. In 1988, German researchers took both water- and alcohol-soluble extracts of *E. angustifolia, E. purpurea,* and *E. pallida* roots and flowering tops. All the extracts promoted phagocytosis after oral administration to mice. For all three species, the alcohol-soluble components stimulated phagocytosis more than did the water-soluble ones. Of the water-soluble constituents, only those from *E. purpurea* showed any activity in these tests (Bauer, Jurck, et al, 1988). This is the first definitive trial comparing the activity of constituents of the three species after the identification of adulteration problems in the mid-1980s cast doubt on previous analytical trials. Before that time, some of what had been tested as *E. angustifolia* was probably *E. pallida,* and some *E. purpurea* samples were probably *Parthenium integrifolium.*

Isobutylamides

If you bite into a root of *Echinacea angustifolia* or *E. purpurea,* you will notice a characteristic tingling sensation in your mouth. This is caused by *isobutylamides,* the most prominent of the alcohol-soluble constituents of echinacea. These substances also promote the flow of saliva. Among herbalists, the intensity and durability of this sensation has come to be an indicator of echinacea quality. This may or may not be accurate, because some products—such as the German *E. purpurea* products, which do not produce this tingling—have been proven in clinical trials to be effective immunostimulants.

A large number of different isobutylamides are present in some echinacea species. Fourteen isobutylamides have been isolated from *E. angustifolia* and eleven from *E. purpurea*. These particular constituents appear only in minute amounts in *E. pallida*. The characteristic chemical structures of the isobutylamides are somewhat different in *E. angustifolia* and *E. purpurea*. Differences in the chemical structures of the isobutylamides between species occur primarily in the roots. The isobutylamides in the leaves of all three species are similar in structure (Bauer and Wagner, 1991). The most important isobutylamide components have the unwieldy name of *dodeca-(2E,4E,8Z,10E/Z)-tetraenoic acid isobutylamides*. The relative content of these components in various parts of the three echinacea species are shown in Table 5.1.

TABLE 5.1   ISOBUTYLAMIDE CONTENT OF SOME ECHINACEA SPECIES (DODECA-(2E,4E,8Z,10E/Z)-TETRAENOIC ACID ISOBUTYLAMIDES)

E. angustifolia root	.009% to .151%
E. angustifolia leaf	negligible
E. purpurea root	.004% to .039%
E. purpurea leaf	.001% to .030%
E. pallida root and leaf	negligible

(Source: Bauer and Wagner, 1991)

Thus, on average, angustifolia roots contain from three to five times as much of the main isobutylamides as purpurea roots or leaves. The relative amounts of these isobutylamides matches the relative reputation of the three roots among North American clinical herbalists: *E. angustifolia* root is the strongest medicine; *E. purpurea* root is not as strong, but nevertheless works therapeutically, perhaps in somewhat higher doses; preparations of *E. purpurea* leaf are also effective; and *E. pallida* is questionable as a medicine. Whether this reputation is accurate will require comparative clinical trials to determine. The reputation of *E. angustifolia* as the "best" species — whether deserved or not — may be based on its average higher content of isobutylamides, which cause stronger tingling and saliva-producing sensations, perhaps only giving the impression of being a stronger medicine.

Echinacea isobutylamides have broad immune-stimulating effects (Bauer and Wagner, 1991). They may also have anti-inflammatory and fever-lowering effects. A 1994 study showed that they inhibited the enzymes cyclooxygenase and lipoxygenase, which promote inflammation and fever (Muller-Jakic et al., 1994). These are the same enzymes that steroids, aspirin, and non-steroidal anti-inflammatory drugs like acetaminophen and ibuprofen inhibit.

Polyacetylenes

Another group of alcohol-soluble constituents called *polyacetylenes* have been found in all three species. Their concentration is highest in the roots. They are considered to be the most important of the alcohol-soluble constituents in *E. pallida*. The presence of certain compounds of this group in

E. pallida is used as a chemical fingerprint to distinguish it from other species for identification.

These compounds may have been important in the plants used by the Native Americans, who used the fresh plants, but they are not likely to be significant constituents in modern commercial preparations because they degrade rapidly. Several researchers have found them to be mostly degraded, and present in only trace amounts, in commercial products (Schulte, 1967; Bauer, Khan, Wagner, 1988). This degradation in storage may be responsible for the poor reputation among herbalists of *E. pallida* as a medicine. It may also explain why the Eclectics, who generally failed to distinguish between *E. angustifolia* and *E. pallida* described a wide variation in the medicinal activity of the plant.

WATER-SOLUBLE CONSTITUENTS

These constituents are present in the fresh plant, fresh plant juice, and teas. They may also be present in the dried plant, but they may degrade to some extent with drying. Depending on their individual characteristics, they may or may not be present in tinctures, which include portions of both alcohol and water. Most of echinacea's water-soluble constituents are not present in commercial products other than raw herb in capsules or tablets. As we saw above, current scientific opinion is that the alcohol-soluble fractions of echinacea are the most important in commercial preparations. Still, a large volume of research has been done on water-soluble constituents, and some of them may play a role in some commercial preparations.

Polysaccharides

By far the most research into plant constituents of echinacea in recent decades has been into the water-soluble *polysaccharides* — huge sugar molecules. Using concentrated and purified extractions of these polysaccharides, scientists have found wide-ranging immune-system-stimulating activity. Some of the actions of these polysaccharides are (Wagner and Proksch, 1981):

- anti-inflammatory activity (cortisone-like)
- increase in antibody production
- increased white blood cell count
- inhibition of hyaluronidase
- protection from radiation damage
- stimulation of antibody-forming cells
- stimulation of cell-mediated immunity
- stimulation of phagocytosis

Almost all of this research has been in the petri dish or in animals, and most of it has used injections, so its relevance to present commercial products is questionable. These polysaccharides are insoluble in alcohol and are not present in tinctures — the form that the Eclectics used to bring echinacea to worldwide fame. They may also be digested before entering the bloodstream if taken orally. Even in the German products made from echinacea juice and low levels of alcohol, polysaccharides are present only in greatly reduced amounts, and what remains in the juice is of a different composition than that found in the purified extractions on which much of the research has been done (Bauer and Wagner, 1991). The erroneous impression that these studies have clinical relevance to forms of echinacea most often used by the public has been responsible for several widely circulated myths.

Wagner and Proksch, who did much of the pioneering echinacea polysaccharide research, also tested polysaccharides from other plants for their ability to stimulate phagocytosis (Wagner and Proksch, 1985). One finding was that polysaccharides from chamomile flowers were as potent immune-system-stimulators as those from echinacea. If such polysaccharides were, in fact, important components of either plant in common medicinal preparations, then we'd expect chamomile to have a reputation as an immune-system-stimulant, which it does not. Immune-system-stimulating effects have also been discovered in the polysaccharides of rice, wheat, bamboo, and sugarcane (Hobbs, 1989), and none of these are noted immune-system-stimulants.

The motivation for the polysaccharide research has been commercial—to develop patentable pharmaceutical immune-system-stimulating drugs—rather than purely academic research casting light on the actions of currently available forms of echinacea. In fact, an industrial process to produce these polysaccharides from cell cultures has been developed in Germany (Wagner, Stuppner, Puhlmann, et al., 1989). We might see them in the future there as prescription injectable drugs.

ARABINOGALACTANS   One particular kind of polysaccharide is called an *arabinogalactan*. This was one of the first polysaccharides to be completely isolated in a purified form from echinacea (Proksch and Wagner, 1987). This compound has attracted the attention of cancer researchers (Luettig et al, 1989) and others (Wagner, Stuppner, Schäfer, and Zenk, 1988), who have found that, when injected into mice, the arabinogalactans increase the secretion of anti-tumor substances.

Arabinogalactan and related arabinogalactan-protein complexes have been found in all three of the common species of echinacea (Beuscher, 1995). Unlike some larger polysaccharides, they are present in some alcohol-soluble products; experiments by Beuscher found them present in 30-percent alcohol extractions of all three species. They may not be present in tinctures with higher alcohol content. We may hear more about arabinogalactans in the future, as immune-system-stimulating constituents of echinacea or as pharmaceutical chemotherapeutic drugs. An industrial process to produce them from echinacea cell cultures has been developed in Germany (Wagner, Stuppner, Puhlmann, et al., 1989).

Arabinogalactans from many other plants are also being investigated as immune-system-stimulants. Arabino-galactans are present in such traditional immune-system-stimulating plants as wild indigo (*Baptisia tinctoria*) and cedar (*Thuja occidentalis*). However, they are also present in carrots, radishes, black beans, pears, corn, wheat, red wine, tomatoes, sorghum, bamboo, coconuts, and milk, so it is questionable whether their mere presence in a plant confers immune-system-stimulating properties or whether they are responsible for immune-system-enhancing effects in common echinacea preparations (D'Adamo, 1996). Their effectiveness as concentrated isolated constituents does not necessarily mean that they are effective in common preparations.

INULIN Echinacea contains a polysaccharide constituent called *inulin*. This constituent is common to several other plants with reputations as "blood cleansers," or tonics, including burdock *(Arctium lappa)*, dandelion root *(Taraxacum officinale)*, and elecampagne *(Inula helenium)*. Some North American writers have stated that inulin is a major immune-system-stimulating constituent of echinacea, but none of the German researchers specializing in echinacea constituents has stated this view.

Cichoric Acid

Several studies have shown that *cichoric acid* — a water-soluble component of *E. purpurea* not found in the other two major species — has strong phagocytosis-stimulating properties (Bauer, Remiger, et al, 1989). Unlike most of the other water-soluble constituents, this one is present in alcoholic tinctures, remaining dissolved in the water portion of the tincture.

Cynarine

Cynarine, which is present in *E. angustifolia* roots, is chemically related to the cichoric acid in *E. purpurea*. It has not been extensively studied, but further research may reveal that it contributes to that species' medicinal effects.

Echinacoside

Echinacoside, which is chemically related to both cichoric acid and cynarine, was once thought to be a significant medicinal constituent of echinacea. This is no longer the case. It was also formerly thought to be unique to the angustifolia species, which has also been disproved (Awang, 1991). Based on these misconceptions, some companies produce products with a standardized echinacoside content. This may be useful to determine that the original product was really echinacea (see Chapter 8), but it won't predict immune-stimulating activity.

Recent research indicates that the three constituents above—cichoric acid, cynarine, and echinacoside—may contribute to wound healing, burn healing, and anti-infective effects of echinacea extracts when they are used topically. Cynarine and echinacoside were found to inhibit hyaluronidase, thickening the extracellular gel and inhibiting infection (Facino et al., 1993).

Cichoric acid, cynarine, and echinacoside were also found to inhibit free-radical damage to collagen, a constituent of the skin. This could indicate protective and/or healing effects on sunburn and other burns (Facino et al., 1995).

TABLE 5.2   THE SUSPECTED ACTIVE CONSTITUENTS IN THREE ECHINACEA SPECIES

	E. angustifolia	E. purpurea	E. pallida
ALCOHOL-SOLUBLE			
isobutylamides	x	x	
polyacetylenes			x
WATER-SOLUBLE			
polysaccharides	x	x	x
arabinogalactan	x	x	x
cichoric acid		x	
cynarine	x		

CONCLUSION

Research into echinacea constituents is by no means complete, and we can expect to see new and revealing information from future research. An area of special relevance to commercial products or to understanding comparative species strength will be research into the pharmacological properties of the isobutylamides in humans.

What we know about echinacea:

- The three most common echinacea species each possess a unique chemical "fingerprint" of constituents. They are three different medicines.
- All three species contain various constituents that are immune-system-stimulating in animal and petri-dish studies.
- The alcohol-soluble constituents are the most important medicinal agents in common commercial echinacea preparations, and those in *E. angustifolia* and *E. purpurea* are the most stable.
- Water-soluble constituents may be more important in injectable echinacea forms and may be promising sources of pharmaceutical immune-system-stimulating drugs.

What we don't know about echinacea is which specific constituents of the various species are most important clinically. Although a wide variety of constituents have been investigated in animal and petri-dish studies, comparative clinical information is non-existent.

CHAPTER 6

CLINICAL
RESEARCH ON
ECHINACEA

*A person who is restricted to laboratory experiments,
especially if he is more or less prejudiced as I was
against echinacea, is not in a position to judge with
discretion. Nor is a laboratory man to be considered
an "authority" in clinical directions . . .*

John Uri Lloyd, apologizing for his
initial rejection of echinacea

The best evidence for the clinical effectiveness of the echinacea species comes from its history of use and from the reports of Eclectic and German physicians and other medical herbalists who use it in their practices. Such evidence does not meet the standards of proof for modern medical science, however, so in this section, I'll describe what we know about echinacea on the basis of scientific study, rather than from medical tradition.

For plants as famous as those in the echinacea genus, so widely used by turn-of-the-century physicians in the U.S. and by contemporary physicians in Germany, surprisingly

little conclusive scientific knowledge of their clinical properties has been gained. In the eighteen years that I've been
using echinacea and reviewing scientific studies and traditional literature about it, prevailing scientific opinions about
the properties of the three species and their active constituents have changed several times, and I suspect they will
change that much again in the next eighteen years.

As we saw in the last chapter, scientists agree that certain constituents in all three of the major commercial species
of echinacea have some level of immune-system-stimulating
properties, but only a handful of human clinical trials using
real-life situations have been undertaken. Most research has
been performed on animals and on cell cultures in petri
dishes, and has been done with isolated and concentrated
constituents of echinacea rather than with whole-plant
preparations such as you would buy in a health food store or
herb shop. Although the research, as a whole, supports the
traditional use of echinacea as an immune-system-stimulant,
we have very little definitive information from scientific trials
about how to use echinacea, what species or plant parts are
most effective, and what form or forms are most useful.

ECHINACEA RESEARCH

Echinacea is one of the most studied of the medicinal herbs,
with about four hundred research papers published on its
constituents, pharmacology, and clinical effects. Most of the
research has been conducted in Germany. With so much
published literature, it is unusual that so little about the clinical effects of its species have been determined according to
scientific standards. The main reasons for weakness of the
clinical evidence are as follows:

- Most of the research has been done on animals and in petri-dish studies. Because the pharmacological dynamics of plants and drugs—how they are similated, transformed, used, and excreted in the body—usually differs widely between animals and humans, human studies have to be done before the relevance of such preliminary studies can be determined. Such research can suggest possible clinical uses, but cannot prove clinical effects.
- Much of the research has been done on isolated echinacea constituents rather than whole-plant extracts. It is possible, and even common, that constituents in low concentration in a plant have no measurable effect at all when taken as part of the plant, even if when isolated and concentrated they have a strong effect.
- Many of the published clinical articles are not controlled trials, but simply practitioner reports. They may provide us with useful information, but they don't prove anything by scientific standards.
- Most published clinical articles have described injectable forms of echinacea, which have some strikingly different properties than the oral forms available to physicians and the public in North America. Constituents that may be highly active in injections may be destroyed or altered by the digestive system or the liver before they enter the general circulation after oral administration.
- Most of the well-designed German clinical trials of the oral use of echinacea have evaluated products in which echinacea is combined with other herbs.

Thus, the actual effect of echinacea itself remains unclear in these trials.

- Much of the research, whether analytical or clinical, prior to 1987, is of questionable value because of the likelihood of adulteration of the "echinacea" used in the trials. See Chapter 8 on adulteration.

For these reasons, in the section that follows I will report only on research that has used echinacea in human trials in the forms in which it is available to the North American public. For a thorough review of all the scientific literature on echinacea, see Bauer and Wagner (1991), Foster (1991), or Hobbs (1990).

White Blood Cell Count

In an early Eclectic study of the effects of echinacea on white blood cell counts, a group of healthy medical students volunteered to take therapeutic doses of echinacea for a period of four days (Ram, 1935). They took an alcohol extract of echinacea (Specific Echinacea, Lloyd Brothers Pharmacy) four times a day for the equivalent of between 520 mg and 4,300 mg per day of *Echinacea angustifolia* root. They took the medicine, dissolved in a larger amount of water, before meals and at bedtime. Blood was drawn before the start of the study and then again at the same time each twenty-four hours. The subjects were not told how much medicine each one was taking, but were asked to describe any changes effected by the drug. I'll review the subjective observations of the students in the section on side effects in Chapter 7.

The daily blood counts showed normal variations among the individuals in the group. In every case, there was a strong increase in white blood cell levels during the first two days. In two-thirds of the cases, the highest count reached was at the end of twenty-four hours' medication. In the remaining third, the peak was reached after forty-eight hours' administration. From the highest point, the counts of the total white blood cells gradually dropped until, on the third and fourth days, they approximated the normal count. The red blood cell count was not significantly altered. The averages of the counts for the entire group are listed in Table 6.1.

The table shows that the total white blood cell count — one measure of the activity of the immune system and the body's response to infection — rose about 30 percent in the first twenty-four hours, declining back to normal within three days. The neutrophils and monocytes, the most important white blood cell types to attack and destroy invading bacteria, viruses, and other toxins, also peaked after about twenty-four hours and were back to normal levels within

TABLE 6.1   INCREASES IN WHITE BLOOD CELL
COUNTS WHILE TAKING *ECHINACEA
ANGUSTIFOLIA* TINCTURE

Period	Total	Neutrophils	Eosinophils	Basophils	Lympho-cytes	Mono-cytes
Start	8,990	5,560	185	83	2,400	451
24 hrs	12,060	9,010	209	105	2,810	592
48 hrs	10,250	5,910	125	111	4,360	591
72 hrs	8,880	5,190	217	88	2,950	376
96 hrs	7,720	5,160	252	74	2,650	399

three days. The lymphocytes, which are important in long-term and organism-specific immunity, peaked at forty-eight hours and came back to normal after four days. The study shows that the body responds to echinacea with a response typical in infection: The cells that indicate general immunity peak first, followed by a peak in organism-specific immunity.

White Blood Cell Activity

The study described above measured only one parameter of overall immunity: the white blood cell count. Another important measure is the activity of those white blood cells. The process by which white blood cells eat invading organisms is called phagocytosis. The white blood cell surrounds and engulfs a bacterium or a virus, which ends up inside the white blood cell. White blood cells, and similar cells throughout the tissues of the body, can have different appetites for bacteria or other debris at different times. Sometimes they are hardly "hungry" or reactive to invaders at all. At other times, they become "ravenously hungry" and, like schools of sharks in a feeding frenzy, quickly eat large amounts of foreign matter.

So the "appetite" of these cells is an important measure of overall immunity at any one time. They are excited to eat by various chemicals produced by other components of the immune system. It is possible that constituents of echinacea mimic these substances or else trigger their secretion, stimulating the white blood cells and macrophages to heightened activity.

Among the first laboratory studies of *Echinacea angustifolia* were those of Dr. Victor Von Unruh around 1915 in New York City (Von Unruh, 1915). Von Unruh treated many tuberculosis patients, and he used a number of them for his experiments with echinacea. Altogether, he drew the blood of more than a hundred patients with infectious diseases, measuring the bacteria-eating power of the white blood cells before and after administering *E. angustifolia*. He describes the result thus:

> *The stimulation toward phagocytosis became very evident in cases where it was impossible to find any evidence of phagocytosis before echinacea was administered, and where after the use of this drug for a period of only a few days, the phagocytes were seen to contain as many as eight bacilli each within the cell.*

(Ellingwood, 1919)

Thus, the white blood cells that previously were suffering from poor appetite gobbled up as many as eight bacteria each within a few days after stimulation by echinacea. In a personal communication with Dr. Finley Ellingwood, an Eclectic professor from the Chicago area, Von Unruh wrote:

> *The [white blood cells] are disinclined to take up bacteria unless they are prepared for phagocytosis by certain substances in the serum that in some manner modifies them. . . . I have definitely demonstrated and am continuing to observe that the action of echinacea on the [white blood cells] is such that it will raise phagocytosis to its possible maximum.*

Von Unruh also found that when the percentage of the white blood cell types that phagocytose bacteria is low, administration of echinacea tends to raise them to a normal level.

A recent study, coming more than seventy years after Von Unruh's work, showed similar results and measured them with precision (Jurcic et al, 1989). Researchers in Germany gave patients oral doses of an alcohol tincture of *E. purpurea* root, such as one might purchase in a health food store today. The test subjects took thirty drops of the tincture three times a day for five days, and a control group took a placebo. Researchers drew the subjects' blood and measured the activity of the phagocytes at the start and at intervals. By day three, phagocytosis in the echinacea group had increased more than forty percent; by day four more than seventy percent, and by day five, 120 percent. Even after the dose was stopped, it was not until day eight that the phagocytosis of the echinacea group fell back into the range of that of the placebo group.

This article is one of the most significant of the recent studies of echinacea, because a companion experiment was done with an injectable form of echinacea. The oral application described above excited the activity of the white blood cells dramatically more than the injections did. Consider for a moment what this implies about the best way to take echinacea. Some constituents of any plant are at least partially digested when taken orally. If it is necessary to get these constituents to a receptor site in the body for them to work, then it would usually be more efficient to inject them, and thus bypass the destruction in the digestive system. Because the opposite effect was shown in this well-designed trial, we can assume that the most important immune-system-stimulating effect of oral doses of echinacea actually happens somewhere *in* the digestive tract, before the ingested echinacea reaches the bloodstream through normal absorption in the intestines.

The most likely candidate for the site of echinacea's action is the lymphatic tissue in the mouth and throat. The rough back part of the tongue, the soft palate at the back of the roof of the mouth, and the tonsils at the sides of the entrance to the throat form a ring of lymphatic tissue that makes up an "early oral warning system" for the body. Like lions guarding a gate, the lymph tissues lying just under the skin here at the entrance to the digestive system absorb and examine a sample of everything that we swallow and anything that makes its way into the mouth. If something foreign or toxic is detected, immune system messages are transmitted rapidly throughout the body through the lymphatic vessels and through the autonomic nervous system.

It is possible that a constituent of echinacea triggers this warning system, perhaps tricking the body into thinking that it is being invaded by a toxic substance and stimulating a massive response. Thus it may be important to *taste* your echinacea and hold it in your mouth for a while to give it maximum contact with the lymphatics in the mouth. This is how the Native Americans used it. Every professional herbalist I have asked believes that liquid forms of echinacea, such as tinctures and fluid extracts, are more effective than dried forms such as capsules or tablets. Perhaps this is because these dried forms keep the powdered herb away from the very tissues it needs to reach in order to stimulate an immune system response. If you want to take capsules or tablets, it may help to open them up or crush them and mix them with a little warm water, then swish the mixture around in your mouth before swallowing it.

Echinacea may also act lower down in the digestive tract. Some substances—such as those in garlic that cause "garlic breath"—are rapidly absorbed through the stomach wall, and this may be the way in which alcohol-soluble echinacea constituents first enter the system. In this case, it is possible that the constituents are transformed in some way by the liver to make them more powerful—an action that is common to many pharmaceutical drugs. Also, tissue similar to the lymphatics and tonsils in the mouth is located throughout the digestive tract, and is especially concentrated near where the small intestine meets the large intestine—in the appendix and in areas known as the Peyer's patches. The best candidates for the site of activity, though, are the mouth and stomach, either of which can explain the relatively rapid response—almost instantaneous—that clinicians see to a large dose of echinacea taken orally.

The stimulation of phagocytosis is one of the most common findings of many of the animal and *in vitro* trials of echinacea, and several different constituents have been isolated from the three species that have this effect in such trials.

Length of Stimulation

We've seen that the number of white blood cells increases for the first few days after taking echinacea before declining toward normal. By then, the activity of the cells has been stimulated. But does the increase of activity offset the decline in the number of cells? What is the overall immune-system-stimulating effect, and how long does it last? One trial using echinacea for prevention of vaginal yeast infections gives us some clues.

In this study (Coeugniet and Kühnast, 1986), a group of 203 women with vaginal candida yeast infections were treated with a conventional antifungal cream (econazol nitrate). They were then divided into five groups. One of the groups received no further treatment. Three of the groups received repeated doses of various injectable forms of echinacea (prescription items in Germany)—under the skin, in the veins, and in the muscles. The fifth group was given a commercial preparation made from the juice of the flowering tops of *E. purpurea*. The groups were then monitored to see how many yeast infections recurred in each. Table 6.2 shows the results.

TABLE 6.2 TREATMENT OF RECURRENT CANDIDA
INFECTION WITH ECHINACEA

Treatment	Number of Patients	Recurrences	Rate of Recurrence (%)
Antifungal cream alone	43	26	60.5
Antifungal cream plus subcutaneous echinacea	20	3	15
Antifungal cream plus intramuscular echinacea	60	3	5
Antifungal cream plus intravenous echinacea	20	3	15
Antifungal cream plus oral echinacea	60	10	16.7

The echinacea treatments, according to these results, increased the patients' resistance to recurring infection. This sort of trial measures overall immune system response independent of its various parts, such as white blood cell count, phagocyte activity, and the many other parameters of the immune system. In order to measure *cell-mediated immunity*, one of the mechanisms of specific immunity I described in detail in Chapter 4, the researchers also administered a standard skin test at the start of the trial, and again after two weeks and ten weeks. The test showed a weakened cell-mediated immunity for the group as a whole at the beginning of the trial. By two weeks, the cell-mediated immunity improved significantly in the groups receiving injections of echinacea. By ten weeks, the group receiving oral echinacea liquid also showed a significant normalization of cell-mediated immunity.

The results of this trial show that the overall immune resistance of the participants receiving echinacea, as measured by rates of recurring infection or by the skin test, continued to improve between weeks two and ten. They also show that the oral echinacea extract, taken for ten weeks, could reach the same level of effectiveness as several of the injectable forms.

Colds and Flu

Two clinical trials on the use of echinacea in colds or flu have been conducted in the last five years, both with positive results, and each yielding useful information about dose or length of treatment.

The first study took 180 volunteers in the first few days of flu-like symptoms or feverish infections of the upper respiratory tract. They were divided into three groups. The first group received a placebo; the second took ninety drops a day of a tincture of *E. purpurea* root (450-mg dose); and the third received 180 drops of the same tincture daily (900-mg dose). The tincture used one part of echinacea by weight in five parts of fifty-five-percent alcohol. The placebo used the same percentage of alcohol with artificial coloring. The patients' symptoms were evaluated after three to four days and then again after eight to ten days. The results showed that ninety drops a day of the tincture was no more effective than the placebo, but 180 drops showed a definite effect, reducing the length and severity of the cold. The superiority of the 180-drop treatment was evident after the measurement at days three to four, and continued to grow through the measurement at days eight to ten.

A second study of echinacea used to treat colds and flu tested the ability of a commercial *E. purpurea* preparation (Echinacin) to prevent recurrences in 108 patients with heightened susceptibility to colds (Schöneberger, 1992). Participants were selected on the basis of having had at least three cold-related infections during the previous winter. Included were such symptoms as ear infection, runny nose, sinus infection, sore throat, laryngitis, bronchitis, pneumonia, swollen glands, and other such signs.

Echinacin is made from the pressed juice of the flowering tops of *E. purpurea,* stabilized with about 22 percent alcohol. This is the same oral product used in the trial on vaginal candida infections described above.

One group of patients received 4 ml—about one tablespoon—of Echinacin twice a day . The other group received a placebo. The groups were monitored after four weeks, and again after eight weeks, to see if participants had contracted colds. Blood tests measuring immune system parameters were also taken at the beginning of the trial and at the two check-in points.

The results of the trial showed that more people in the echinacea group remained infection-free, and the group as a whole had fewer infections, although the results did not reach the level that would constitute statistical proof according to scientific standards. The participants in the echinacea group also tended to have milder infections and went a longer period of time until their first infection—forty days for the echinacea group versus twenty-five days for the placebo group. In the echinacea group, fewer of the infections spread to the lower respiratory tract, resulting in fewer cases of bronchitis. Note that this trial describes both prevention and treatment of colds, because participants continued to take the echinacea when they became infected, with positive results on the severity of the illness.

The researchers analyzed their data and found that one subset of the participants were benefited by the echinacea more than others. These were participants with weakened cell-mediated immunity. Such immunity is measured by the ratio of various T-cells in the body. When the number of T-4 cells drops relative to the number of T-8 cells, an individual is considered to have weakened immunity. This is one of the ways of measuring the progression of HIV infection toward AIDS, for instance. Of the participants in the study who had low T-4 to T-8 ratios (less than 3:2), echinacea was even more effective than it had been in the general group. For these patients, echinacea reduced the severity of infections even more dramatically and also reduced the length of the infections from 7.5 days to 5.3 days, an effect not seen in the larger group.

These two trials are even more important than the first ones described, because these show actual curative or preventive effects, rather than simple improvement in immune system parameters. The first studies show an increase in white blood cell levels and the activity of phagocytes, while these studies show that such increases, as well as other possible effects on the immune system not studied, are enough to actually prevent or favorably treat a medical condition. The trials show that echinacea may be taken for several months at a time while still showing immune system stimulation.

Other Research

The research described above is the most relevant to the human clinical use of echinacea. Other published research, although less conclusive from a clinical point of view, is nevertheless interesting, so I'll describe some of it briefly.

TOPICAL USE OF ECHINACEA   We saw in Chapters 2 and 3 that Native Americans and Eclectic physicians both used echinacea topically, for infected wounds, swellings, inflammations, and other skin conditions. Echinacea is used this way in Germany today, where a topical product is in common use by physicians. The Eclectics diluted their echinacea tinctures with six parts of water before applying them to the skin. The German product uses about the same percentage of echinacea juice in its ointment.

In a large-scale review of 4,598 clinical cases, Viehmann (1978) concluded that the ointment was a highly effective treatment for a variety of skin conditions. The review included 1,453 patients with wounds, 900 with varicose ulcers, 628 with eczema, 626 with burns, 222 with herpes simplex, and 212 with inflammatory skin conditions. Treatment of wounds, burns, and herpes infections gave the best results, with better than a ninety-percent positive response. Treatment of varicose ulcers was least effective, with about a seventy-percent response—an excellent cure rate for a condition that, unlike the others, does not easily heal on its own. This was not a controlled trial, so it does not "prove" that echinacea works. It does, however, reflect common medical practice in Germany, and tends to verify the earlier uses by Native Americans and Eclectic doctors.

This echinacea ointment has also been used in Germany to treat psoriasis (Kortung and Born, 1954; Kortung and Rasp, 1954) and pemphigus (Schnursbusch, 1955). Other researchers have treated psoriasis with conventional topical preparations and oral echinacea extracts (Gaertner, 1968).

The mechanisms for action of the topical preparations appear to be through promotion of the regeneration of tissue, reduction of inflammation, and promotion of local immune system reactions (Foster, 1991). Oral preparations do not necessarily have the same tissue-strengthening or anti-inflammatory effects.

ECHINACEA INJECTIONS   Most of the clinical studies published in Germany on echinacea have been done with injectable forms, either in the veins, under the skin, or in the muscles of the patients. The German injectable products are made from the juice of the flowering tops of *E. purpurea*, stabilized, sterilized, and filtered according to pharmaceutical standards, and monitored for contamination. Once, after publishing an article mentioning the German use of injectable forms of echinacea, I received a letter asking if the writer could safely inject an echinacea tincture. The answer is categorically "No!" Abscesses and serious infections can result from the injection of unsterilized and unfiltered plant material.

Numerous conditions have been treated in Germany with echinacea injections. Many of the reports, although published in scientific and medical journals, do not meet scientific standards for controlled trials. However, they reflect the way that physicians in Germany use injectable forms of echinacea. These treatments are presently not legal in the U.S.

Some of the conditions that have been treated with injectable forms of echinacea with positive results are (Bauer and Wagner, 1991; Foster, 1991, Hobbs, 1990).

allergies
arthritis
bronchitis
ear infection
eczema
frostbite
gunshot wounds
gynecological infections
infections
influenza
pelvic inflammatory disease
prostatitis
psoriasis
skin ulcers
tonsillitis
tuberculosis

urinary tract infections
warts
whooping cough
wound healing

The differences between the oral and injectable routes of administration of any medicine can be profound, and these differences may be even stronger than usual for echinacea. A substance injected into the veins of the body, bypassing all normal defense mechanisms, is rapidly circulated throughout the body, normally reaching the distant parts of the body in a matter of seconds. The route for substances of large molecular weight injected into the muscles or under the skin is slightly different because they must make their way through the lymphatic vessels and nodes before entering the general circulation. With either method, an injection bypasses the normal barrier defenses of the immune system (see Chapter 4) and may be quickly circulated more or less intact throughout the body.

Substances taken orally, on the other hand, must run the gauntlet of digestive juices — saliva, stomach acid, and intestinal and pancreatic digestive enzymes — before they are assimilated. Even then, once absorbed in the intestine, they are circulated through the liver before they can enter the general circulation. The liver, which specializes in screening out foreign matter and chemically transforming potentially toxic substances, will not necessarily let drugs or herbal constituents pass unchanged, if at all.

Many differences exist in the clinical effects of oral and injectable echinacea forms, and these are summarized in Table 6.3. One of the most notable is that fever reactions are common with echinacea injections. A temperature rise of one or two degrees Fahrenheit occurs in most patients. Such a rise is not considered a problem by German practitioners, who view it as a healthy healing response, possibly related to enhanced immune system activity (Bauer and Wagner, 1991). Another reaction to injections is stimulation of the adrenal glands. These glands normally respond to stress by secreting anti-inflammatory hormones similar to synthetic immune-system-suppressing cortisone medications. The shock of sudden injection of echinacea plant material appears to trigger this response, which has not been observed with oral use in either animals or humans.

TABLE 6.3   SOME DIFFERENCES BETWEEN INJECTABLE AND ORAL FORMS OF ECHINACEA

Injectable	Oral
Illegal in North America	Legal in North America
Fever reaction common	Fever reaction rare
Stimulates a stress response from the adrenal glands	No stress response
Can cause immune system suppression	No immune system suppression noted
Anti-inflammatory	No evidence for this
Eosinophils lowered by up to 50%	No evidence of lowering
Contraindicated in pregnancy	No such contraindication
Fast effect on cell-mediated immunity	Slow effect
Weaker effect on phagocytosis	Stronger effect
Stimulates properdin-complement system	No evidence of effect

The observation of immune system suppression in several trials using injections (Coeugniet and Elek, 1987; Jurcic et al, 1989) was the source of inaccurate rumors that oral echinacea might have this effect. Similar immunosuppression, characterized by a decline in the T-4:T-8 lymphocyte ratio and lasting for about the same length of time, has been observed with injections accompanying various immunizations (Brody et al., 1964; Eibl et al., 1984; Siegel et al., 1981). Injections of echinacea at the rate of about one a week do not appear to have this effect, while more freequent injections do. The clinical trial in vaginal candidiasis described above showed a normalization rather than a suppression of the cell-mediated immune system with once-a-week injections.

One of the reasons for the differences observed between these two routes of administration may be the presence of polysaccharides in the echinacea juice commonly used in injections in Germany. Polysaccharides are among the most intensely studied constituents of echinacea (see Chapter 5). These large sugar molecules may be digested by the human body, like any other starches or sugars, and reduced to glucose before they can enter the general circulation. Some polysaccharides, such as the *acemannan* in aloe vera juice, are only absorbed at a rate of one percent (McAnalley and McDaniel, 1993). Thus they could reach the bloodstream in the injectable forms at one hundred times the level they do with oral use, even with consumption of the raw plant material or by drinking the juice. As we noted in Chapter 5, polysaccharides are insoluble in alcohol, are not present in alcohol tinctures, and are present only in greatly reduced amounts even with the amount of alcohol used to stabilize German oral echinacea juice products.

Injections of polysaccharides in animal trials have been found to induce the secretion of substances from immune system cells that trigger a fever (Luettig et al, 1989), and other polysaccharides and glycoproteins similar to those found in injectable forms of echinacea are known to evoke fever reactions (Bauer and Wagner, 1991). Thus, their delivery in injectable forms may explain most of the differences in reactions between injections and oral use.

TRIALS WITH COMBINATION PRODUCTS   Some of the best-designed German clinical research into the oral use of echinacea investigated products that combined echinacea with other immune-system-stimulating herbs. Any beneficial clinical effect could have been due to any of the herbs, or to a synergy of their effects, rather than simply to echinacea. One product—Esberitox—combines echinacea with *Baptisia tinctoria* (wild indigo) and *Thuja occidentalis* (white cedar). These two powerful herbs, which can have quite unpleasant side effects, are generally not available to the public in North America, so reproduction of the formula would be difficult here. Such combinations were shown to be effective in the following conditions (Bauer and Wagner, 1991; Foster, 1991; Hobbs, 1990):

- healing bacterial skin infections
- increasing the phagocytic activity of macrophage cells
- prevention and therapy for upper respiratory tract infections
- prevention for colds and influenza
- protection from the white blood cell count drop that often accompanies radiation therapy

- therapy for influenza
- urogenital infections

Animal trials published in 1991 demonstrate that such combination products are more effective than echinacea alone (Wagner and Jurcic, 1991). Phagocytosis was measured after administration to mice of *E. angustifolia* tincture and two other echinacea extracts, and with various combinations of *E. angustifolia* with *Eupatorium perfoliatum* (boneset), *Baptisia tinctoria* (wild indigo), and *Arnica montana* (leopard's bane). Arnica, which can be toxic, was in homeopathic dilution. Phagocytosis was stimulated progressively as constituents of the formula were added. The combination product reached a maximum stimulation of about 50 percent over that of *E. angustifolia* alone. Because the combination products are more effective than echinacea alone, the clinical trials do not demonstrate clinical effectiveness of echinacea. The additive effects of the other herbs, from a scientific point of view, could have pushed the combination over the threshold of effectiveness.

HOMEOPATHIC DILUTIONS Limited research has also been done with homeopathic preparations used on animals, and immune-system-stimulating activity was demonstrated at dilutions of 1:100, 1:10,000, and 1:100,000,000. Bauer and Wagner state: "It can be concluded that a clear distinction between the two types of preparation for the purposes of immunostimulation is not possible at present and is perhaps unnecessary (Bauer and Wagner, 1991).

HYALURONIC ACID Some research has shown that echinacea constituents may have anti-hyaluronidase activity. As mentioned in Chapter 4, hyaluronidase interacts with hyaluronic acid in the tissues to maintain a gel-like substance in the intercellular spaces. If this gel becomes thicker, it presents a greater barrier to the spread of bacteria and viruses. Some bacteria, including the streptococcus that accompanies sore throats, produce their own hyaluronidase in order to move through this gel. Echinacea seems to counter this effect and to strengthen the gel, especially with injectable and topical applications (Koch, 1952, 1953); this could be an important contributor to echinacea's wound-healing ability. There is no research showing this effect with oral use.

CONCLUSION

Echinacea research—both clinical investigations and studies of its constituents—supports the traditional use of echinacea as an immune-system stimulant, anti-inflammatory, and wound-healing agent. Well-designed clinical trials, however, have been rare; the two best-designed ones came only in the last five years.

What we know:

- Extracts of echinacea, taken orally, raise the white blood cell count for a few days.
- Extracts increase the activity of the non-specific defense system including the activity of phagocytes, the cells that "eat" foreign particles, bacteria, viruses, and cell debris,
- Extracts also normalize cell-mediated immunity, which is important in fighting viral infections and tumors.
- Because they activate both non-specific and cell-mediated immunity, extracts are potentially useful in almost any infective process.

- Topical applications have anti-inflammatory, immune-system-stimulating, and wound-healing properties.
- Science has not demonstrated which species of echinacea, if any, is superior in clinical applications for the human being. There is a temptation to apply animal and *in vitro* trials to answer this question, but this is not appropriate without comparative human clinical trials.

CHAPTER 7

CAUTIONS, CONTRAINDICATIONS, AND SIDE EFFECTS

An adage of ancient Greek medicine holds as true today as it did 2,500 years ago: "Above all, do no harm." In recent decades, we are experiencing a renewal of clinical herbalism in the U.S. because plant medicines in general do less harm than pharmaceutical medicines do. People are seeking herbs as medicines because they are less toxic and have fewer side effects than drugs.

But plants are not completely harmless. Even though they are less likely to be toxic—causing physical harm or death—herbs that are strong enough to act as medicines can also produce side effects. These side effects may cause pain or discomfort. Unfortunately, when such side effects occur, individuals with a romantic notion about herbs imagine that they are "healing crises" or even that they are unrelated to the herbs. Of the medicinal herbs available to the public in North America today, echinacea is one of the least toxic, and also among the least likely to cause side effects. It can produce side effects, however, in larger doses and with longer use.

TOXICITY

Researchers have been unable to identify any outright toxicity in echinacea extracts. Formal toxicity trials of echinacea were not published before 1991, but unpublished industry reports starting in 1976 are reported by Hobbs (1990). Various isolated polysaccharides from echinacea cell cultures were found to be non-toxic in 1989 in standard tests (Lenk, 1989; Schimmer et al, 1989). In 1991, German researchers gave both oral and intravenous doses of *E. purpurea* juice to rats and mice in huge quantities—larger than a human being could practically ingest—for four weeks and found no toxicity or potential carcinogenicity in a panel of standard tests (Mengs et al, 1991).

German Press Reports

The German magazine *Die Zeit* reported in May 1996, that three fatalities have occurred due to allergic reactions to echinacea (Hansen, 1996). The article was sensationalist, and also claimed that echinacea has no medicinal effects other than a placebo effect. Resulting television coverage broadcast the claim throughout Germany, and you may one day read the rumor in North American media. Dr. Rudi Bauer, one of the world's leading echinacea researchers, published a rebuttal to the article in the scientific journal *Zeit-*

schrift für Phytotherapie (Bauer, 1996). Bauer reviewed the cases and asserts that no causal effect was demonstrated between the use of echinacea and the fatalities. He notes that a German regulatory commission also reviewed the cases and found no reason to take action to restrict echinacea availability in Germany. Bauer also points out that more than ten million units of echinacea are sold annually in Germany, and that if any substantial risk of fatal allergic reactions exists, then more cases would have been reported.

CONTRAINDICATIONS

We have no contraindications handed down to us from traditional use. A German regulatory commission has suggested several contraindications, however. The official German echinacea monograph offers no contraindications for external use of echinacea, but states that other applications are contraindicated in "progressive systemic diseases like tuberculosis, leukosis, collagen disorders, or multiple sclerosis." This would theoretically include autoimmune disorders such as systemic lupus or rheumatoid arthritis, although they are not mentioned by name. Multiple sclerosis is suspected to have an autoimmune component in which the immune system attacks the sheath that encases the nerves. Leukosis is abnormal proliferation of the white blood cells or the tissues that produce them, and includes diseases like leukemia. The reasoning here is that if the disease is due to overactivity or imbalance of the immune or collagen-making systems, then it does not make sense to stimulate them. The commission also lists contraindications for injectable forms of echinacea in diabetes or pregnancy.

Autoimmunity

In ten years of searching scientific literature and interviewing both physicians and scientists on the issue, I've been unable to find a single case or even a rumor of a case in which echinacea *in oral doses* made any of the above-named conditions worse. This is especially true in autoimmune diseases. I've personally provided long-term care to patients with lupus, and I've interviewed a naturopathic physician who has lupus herself, and in each case the individual was able to use echinacea for normal transient surface infections with no stimulation or exacerbation of their lupus symptoms (Bergner, 1990).

One theory of autoimmune disease is that it can arise not simply from an immune system that is too strong, but from one that is overwhelmed or too weak. Certain bacteria—some of them natural residents of the intestines—have proteins in their cell walls that are similar to proteins found in various human tissues. If these bacteria are present in a chronic infection in the body, perhaps from lesions in the intestinal wall that allow them into the bloodstream, and the body does not handle the infection quickly, the antibodies the body makes against them may attack the corresponding human tissue as well (Pizzorno, 1996). The Chinese military philosopher Sun Tsu stated that "Nobody ever benefited from protracted warfare," and the adage applies to infection as well. An inefficient response to such bacteria may end up spreading the "war" to the body's own tissues. According to this theory, a stimulation of the immune system could give it the boost necessary to "win" the war, thus cooling off the systemic or local inflammation that is causing the symptoms of the autoimmune disease.

TABLE 7.1   KNOWN BACTERIA THAT CAN
             TRIGGER AUTOIMMUNE DISEASES

Microorganism	Disease
Campylobacter	Reiter's syndrome
Candida albicans	irritable bowel syndrome
Escherichia coli-diabetes	mellitus, myasthenia gravis
Klebsiella pneumoniae	myasthenia gravis
Proteus vulgaris	myasthenia gravis
Salmonella	Reiter's syndrome
Shigella	Reiter's syndrome
Yersinia enterococolitica	arthritis, Graves' disease, Hashimoto's disease, Reiter's syndrome, iritis

(Source: Pizzorno, 1996)

This theoretical use for echinacea is unproven, but published clinical reports in Germany have indicated that echinacea can be an effective treatment for the autoimmune rheumatoid arthritis (Meissner, 1950a, 1950b, 1951; Schuster, 1952, Reuss, 1979). Note that these physicians used injectable forms of echinacea, and closely monitored the patients. Self-treatment of rheumatoid arthritis with large doses, or long-term application, may still be inappropriate.

Tuberculosis

Tuberculosis is not a simple infection. In complicated cases, the patient's own immune system destroys lung tissue in a process similar to autoimmunity, perhaps explaining the caution of the German commission. Tuberculosis is usually passed through coughing. Bits of bacteria, suspended in droplets of mucus, linger in the air, especially in crowded living conditions. When they are taken into the lung they are treated like any other invader; the macrophages in the lung eat them. In some instances, tuberculosis may be stronger than the macrophages and may actually take up residence inside a macrophage, reproducing inside it and turning it into a little tuberculosis-breeding factory. The macrophage bursts after a while, releasing hundreds of newly born tuberculosis germs into the lung. More macrophages are attracted to the site to eat these additional bacteria. The disease can stabilize at this point, with the macrophages winning the battle.

If the macrophages have attracted the attention of a wandering T-cell from the bloodstream, however, another chain of events ensues. The T-cell finds the remains of macrophage-eaten tuberculosis germs and secretes chemicals that attract more macrophages to the site and stimulate the local macrophages to a feeding frenzy. As we saw in Chapter 4, macrophages activated in this way may increase their ability to ingest germs by a power of one hundred. These activated macrophages cause scar tissue to form around the area, walling it off from the rest of the body. They also send fever-inducing chemical messages to the brain. At this point, again, the immune system may win the battle and defeat the invading tuberculosis.

If not, however, progressed tuberculosis can become a nightmare. The T-cells eventually recognize that tuberculosis germs are "hiding out" inside the macrophages and begin killing off the infected macrophages. This releases even more germs into the surrounding tissues where they now take up residence in the cells of the lung. The T-cells then begin destroying the infected lung tissue. This stage of the disease is called "liquefaction and cavitation"; portions of the lung are literally liquefied by the immune system's response to the infection, similar to the reaction that causes the body to reject organ transplants. At this point, most of the destruction is coming from the immune system rather than from the tuberculosis infection, and it is a valid question whether to stimulate immunity or not.

However, clinical reports do not show a worsening of tuberculosis at any stage with echinacea treatment. In fact, echinacea seems to be an effective therapy, either alone or as an adjunct to conventional treatments. We saw in Chapter 6 that among the first published echinacea research was that of Dr. Victor Von Unruh of New York, who used echinacea to treat tuberculosis patients. He reported normalization of the body temperature, increase in phagocytosis, destruction of the tuberculosis germs, and shorter duration or stabilization of the disease (Von Unruh, 1915).

German clinicians Heesen and Schroeder have also used echinacea as adjunct therapy in tuberculosis (Heesen and Schroeder, 1960; Heesen, 1964) and report that overall health and X-ray findings improved in a group of several hundred tuberculosis patients receiving echinacea, especially among those with therapy-resistant progressive tuberculosis. The German commission's decision to list a contraindication for echinacea in tuberculosis seems to overlook these clinical reports. They may have felt that the clinical reports did not carry the weight of well-designed clinical trials, or the decision may have been intended to protect the public from self-medication without proper supervision.

It is my opinion that the above conditions should not preclude the use of echinacea for a few weeks to treat a temporary infection. I agree with the commission, however, that someone with these autoimmune conditions should not take echinacea over the long term or in high doses, and that echinacea is not an appropriate treatment for these conditions without careful medical supervision by a physician well-trained in botanical medicine who can order laboratory analyses to monitor the status of the disease.

Leukemia

The German commission's listed contraindication in leukemia and related diseases is likely based on the ability of echinacea to cause a proliferation of the white blood cells. Since these diseases are characterized by elevated white blood cells, it seems prudent caution not to stimulate their growth. The immune system is quite complex, however, with its own internal balancing mechanisms. Echinacea acts on many areas of the system, not just on white blood cells, and it elevates white blood cell count for only a few days. David McLeod, naturopathic doctor, herbalist, and president of the National Herbalists Association of Australia has reported a case study of long-term echinacea use in a patient with leukemia (McLeod 1996a). Leukemia is a cancer of the bone marrow. The majority of patients who die do so from infections because of their weakened immune system. McLeod treated a sixty-eight-year-old leukemia patient for eighteen months, using mainly herbal treatments. The patient took half an ounce a day of each of two remedies, one a combination of immunomodulating herbs, which was adjusted from time to time during the course of treatment, and the other a strong tincture of *Echinacea angustifolia*. An M.D. hematologist monitored blood status every three months. At the beginning of treatment, the patient's white blood cell count was 11.8, with the normal range being between 4.0 and 10.5. After six months, the count was 13.2. By eighteen months, however, the white blood cell count had fallen into the normal range, and it has remained there ever since (McLeod 1996b). The patient's platelet count, another measure of the progression of leukemia, also returned to the normal range. I don't suggest that echinacea "cured" the leukemia, because many herbs were administered in the other formulas. But this patient took about a half ounce of a strong echinacea preparation for more than a year and a half, and it certainly had no adverse effect on his leukemia.

AIDS

A debate has gone back and forth in herbal circles in the U.S. for at least the last ten years about whether echinacea is contraindicated in HIV infection or AIDS. As with the German contraindications, I've been unable to locate a single case in which AIDS was made worse through the use of echinacea, even though AIDS patients commonly take echinacea (Kassler et al, 1991; Gowen et al, 1993). Like the contraindications suggested by the German drug commission, objections to the use of echinacea in AIDS have been theoretical, not based on scientific evidence.

T-4 CELL LEVELS   I was partly responsible for spreading the rumor that AIDS patients should avoid taking echinacea when I stated such a contraindication in an article in *East-West* magazine in August 1988. My reasoning was based on a just-published article showing that echinacea administration could lower T-4 cell counts, with T-8 cell levels remaining stable (Gaisbauer and Zimmerman, 1986). Since AIDS is characterized by a decline in T-4:T-8 cell ratios, it seemed reasonable to avoid echinacea.

Further examination, however, shows that this trial was made with daily injections for seven days, rather than oral use. It is now well-known that frequently repeated injections have this effect, although it has not been noted with oral use. In fact, one clinical trial showed a steady improvement in cell-mediated immunity over a period of ten weeks with oral echinacea administration (Coeugniet and Künast, 1986). Another trial showed that oral echinacea was more effective at preventing infections in those with low T-4:T-8 ratios than in those with normal ratios (Schöneberger, 1992). See my discussion of injectable echinacea in Chapter 6. There is no evidence of any need to avoid the oral use of echinacea to maintain T-4 cell levels.

AUTOIMMUNITY AND AIDS   The second theoretical objection to using echinacea in AIDS comes because AIDS may have an autoimmune component. In the 1990s, the theory emerged among leading AIDS researchers that the HIV virus initiated a series of events that left parts of the immune system attacking itself. So the objection is that immune system stimulation by echinacea could hasten this autoimmune attack. The reasoning is the same as that of the German drug commission.

This autoimmune component of AIDS no longer plays a prominent role in the theory of the dynamics of the disease. Current opinion is that viral replication in massive amounts is countered by similar high production of T-cells, until gradually, usually over years, the virus wins the battle (Wei, 1995). The declining number of T-cells leaves the immune system fatally weakened. If this dynamic is indeed an accurate description, there would be no theoretical reason to avoid echinacea.

TUMOR-NECROSIS-FACTOR   The final objection to the use of echinacea in treating AIDS patients is quite convoluted, but has become widespread in herbal circles in the U.S. in the last few years. It is based on research showing that echinacea polysaccharides increased the secretion of a substance called tumor-necrosis-factor-alpha (TNF-alpha) in animals (Roesler et al, 1991a,b). Some research has shown that a rise in TNF-alpha levels is associated with increased replication of HIV as well as wasting syndrome in the later stages of AIDS.

Although the causal nature of the relationship between TNF-alpha and AIDS progression has not been proven, the weakness of this entire argument lies in the form of "echinacea" that was used in the trial. It was not "echinacea" at all, but rather purified polysaccharides derived from *E. purpurea* cells engineered in the laboratory. These were injected into mice. As we saw in Chapter 5, these polysaccharides, being insoluble in alcohol, are not present in most commercial products. In Chapter 6, I explained the difference in the dynamics of injection versus oral use. Thus, if this trial says anything, it says that you should use caution before injecting concentrated echinacea polysaccharides if you have AIDS. Subsequent research has demonstrated that echinacea tincture, taken orally for four weeks, had no effect on tumor-necrosis-factor in humans (Elsasser-Beile et al., 1996).

Finally, the clinical trial by Schöneberger that I discussed in Chapter 6 showed that echinacea, taken orally, most benefited patients with lowered T4:T8 cell ratios—the same profile as the AIDS patient. Of course, this does not prove anything about contraindication, but it hints that, in the absence of any evidence for contraindication, echinacea *might* in fact be helpful for transient opportunistic infections in AIDS.

IS ECHINACEA IMMUNOSUPPRESSIVE OVER TIME?

Another controversy among North American herbalists is whether echinacea loses it potency after several weeks, or in fact becomes immunosuppressive if taken for too long. The official German regulatory commission for herbal medicines says that echinacea should not be taken for longer than eight weeks. As with the above contraindications, there seems to be no clinical evidence that oral doses of echinacea lose their ability to stimulate the immune system, or that they become immunosuppressive over time. In fact, clinical data shows the opposite. Clinical trials by Coeugniet and Schöneberger (1986) lasted ten and eight weeks, respectively. Each measured the immune system parameters of the participants. The Coeugniet trial showed steadily increasing immunity between weeks two and ten. Schöneberger did not report on immunity, but measured it at the eight-week endpoint of the trial, and presumably would have noted any decline. In other work, Coeugniet and Jurcic found suggestions that echinacea injections, if repeated too frequently, may cause an initial depression of immune system response. Coeugniet and Elek (1987) found, however, that this depression was followed by a rise above the initial levels upon discontinuation of the injections.

Herbal traditions and modern case studies also contradict the idea that echinacea becomes immunosuppressive over time. The Eclectics report using it daily for as long as nine months with no ill effects (Ellingwood, 1919). A German medical text by R.F. Weiss, M.D., known as the "grandfather of phytotherapy" in Germany, says that oral doses of echinacea "should be continued for many weeks and even months, if necessary, even for years. This is inevitable with many chronic conditions where physical resistance has been reduced" (Weiss, 1988). Weiss also states that, even though the exact chemistry of its action is not known, echinacea can be taken anyway because it "certainly can do no harm."

It is the practice of herbalists in Australia to give large doses—up to half an ounce a day—of echinacea to patients for long periods of time, sometimes more than a year (Bone, 1995; McLeod 1996a; McLeod et al., 1996). In several long-term clinical observations, no ill effects were seen in measurement of liver function (McLeod et al., 1996) or immune status (McLeod, 1996a).

CAUTIONS WITH HABITUAL USE

Now that I've shown that there is no evidence that echinacea is immunosuppressive over time, let me state that I think echinacea is one of the most overused and most abused herbs in the U.S. today, and that people who use it too much are harming their health. In Chapter 10, I will go into detail about the lifestyle factors that tend to cause weakened immunity. For now, I will just say that most people who have depressed immunity (including every patient I've met who was taking echinacea habitually) need to change their eating patterns, sleep habits, stress levels, exercise, and/or degree of substance abuse. Frequent colds or infections are nature's way of nudging you in this direction.

If you start to "come down" with a cold or flu, nature is advising you to call in sick at work, get a baby-sitter for the children, stop eating, drink plenty of liquids, take a hot bath, get a good book or video, and go to bed. I'll describe in Chapter 10 how each of these not only helps to fight infection directly, but is also immunorestorative, cleansing the body and rebuilding the immunity in the body at every level. Yes, you may be able to take a large dose of echinacea and "abort" the cold, but echinacea will not make up for the bed rest, reduced stress, fasting, and self-nurturing that your body is asking for.

This is not just a theoretical argument. I know of a doctor in England—a leader in the alternative medicine movement there—who believes that he gave himself a serious case of chronic fatigue by using echinacea to drive away every cold, flu, and infection that came his way, allowing him to go deeper into an unnaturally stressful lifestyle. A patient of my own, with a very stressful lifestyle, did the same thing for more than a year. Eventually she had an extremely painful urinary tract infection that nothing would help—neither antibiotics nor natural treatments—until she finally paid the piper, took time off work, quit drinking coffee, and got some balance in her life. Another woman would have seemed an ideal candidate for echinacea. She had frequent colds and infections, especially vaginal yeast infections. She took echinacea for these with some limited success, but the cause of her depressed immunity was eight continuous years of using birth control pills. Her overall condition continued to erode, in spite of the echinacea, until she stopped taking the pills.

In each of these cases, we can't say that echinacea itself was immunosuppressive. The factors in the lifestyle were causing the problem, not the echinacea. But echinacea use allowed the immune system depression to progress to a more serious level by temporarily masking the real cause of the problem. I recommend that anyone with an infection that lasts longer than a week, or who has more than two colds or cases of the flu in a year, or who has any other frequent infection or sign of immune system depression, see a practitioner of natural medicine for a lifestyle tune-up rather than postponing the inevitable consequences by using echinacea. In some cases, a more serious underlying illness that requires proper diagnosis will be found to be responsible for the weakness.

SIDE EFFECTS

Echinacea can produce minor side effects in the medicinal doses normally taken. Somewhat more serious effects can occur with excessive doses or prolonged use.

In the article by Ram described in Chapter 6, the medical student subjects of the study made notes of the side effects they experienced. They fall into the following categories:

Taste and Smell

Echinacea taken in water had an acrid and slightly nauseating taste. Nausea was more pronounced with the larger doses (650 to 780 mg). Belching followed these larger doses for ten to fifteen minutes, with the gas smelling of echinacea.

Gastrointestinal Symptoms

Doses of 130 to 260 mg produced no gastrointestinal side effects. Larger doses of 650 to 975 mg caused, besides the belching already mentioned, distention of the stomach and a strong secretion of saliva. Eating food relieved these symptoms, but, when the echinacea was taken without food at bedtime, some distress lasted for about an hour.

Echinacea also has a slight laxative effect in doses of about 500 to 1,000 mg. In one constipated subject, a normal bowel movement followed taking echinacea; in a normal subject, fluid stools were produced. These gastrointestinal effects disappeared after forty-eight hours, even with the larger doses.

Genitourinary Symptoms

Echinacea produced a slight diuretic effect, causing more frequent urination with smaller amounts of urine at each attempt. This was evident in all dose ranges, and began to decline after the first two days.

Contemporary Clinical Observations

In the Schöneberger cold-and-flu trial described in Chapter 6, side effects were carefully observed. Remember that these subjects took *E. purpurea* juice (Echinacin) for eight weeks. Eleven of the fifty-four patients taking echinacea reported side effects, including gas, nausea, constipation, tiredness, drowsiness, and headaches.

Topical use may occasionally cause unpleasant effects. In a review of 4,598 clinical cases, Viehmann (1978) reported that 2.3 percent of patients reported side effects to an *E. purpurea* ointment. The patients reported burning pain or intensified itching. Note that alcohol preparations may also irritate the skin in some conditions.

A researcher from Goethe University in Frankfurt, Germany, recently conducted a review of all published and unpublished clinical trials (solicited from researchers) that may have reported echinacea toxicity or side effects. His results included a review of observations of more than 2,000 patients over a period of more than forty years. He found that oral use of echinacea resulted in no more serious side effects than unpleasant taste or mild digestive symptoms (Parnham, 1996).

Ellingwood and the Eclectics' Observations

Dr. Finley Ellingwood was among the most scientific of the Eclectic doctors. Because some modern authors insist that echinacea has no side effects, I will quote his observations directly.

When a half a teaspoonful dose of the tincture is taken into the mouth, a pungent warmth is at once experienced which increases to a tingling, and remains for half an hour after the agent is ejected. If a small quantity be swallowed undiluted, it produces an apparent constriction of the throat, sensation of irritation, and strangulation, much greater in some patients than in others, and always disagreeable.

*The sensation persists for some minutes, notwith-
standing the throat is gargled, water is drunk, and
the agent entirely removed.*

*The toxic effect of this agent is manifested by reduc-
tion of temperature, the frequency of the pulse is diminished, the mucous membrane becomes dry and
parched, accompanied with a prickly sensation; there
is headache of a bursting character, and a tendency to
fainting is observed if the patient assumes an erect
posture. After poisonous doses, these symptoms are
more intensified, the face and upper portion of the
trunk are flushed, there is pain throughout the body,
which is more marked in the large articulations
[joints]. There is dimness of vision, intense thirst,
gastric pains followed by vomiting and watery diarrhea. No fatal case of poisoning is recorded, to our
knowledge, and only when given in extreme doses are
any of the above undesirable influences observed.*

(Ellingwood, 1919)

Dr. Harvey Felter noted that suppression of urination
can occur as a side effect under diseased conditions. He, like
Ellingwood, concludes that in normal medicinal doses no seriously unpleasant symptoms occur, and that no cases of fatal
poisoning in human beings have been recorded at any dose.

THE HOMEOPATHS   In the homeopathic school of medicine, a specially prepared diluted remedy is given to cure the
symptoms that it would cause if given in regular doses or

overdoses. The homeopaths have a variety of ways of gathering their information about toxic symptoms. The data on toxicity may be collected from accidental or deliberate overdoses, or from commonly observed side effects to medical drugs. Much of the early homeopathic information on echinacea was collected from the observations of the Eclectics. Homeopaths also commonly conduct "provings," in which, while in normal health, they take the medicine and see what symptoms appear. Sometimes they take the medicine in normal or toxic doses during a proving, and sometimes they take it in a diluted and homeopathically "potentized" form. At least one such "proving" has been done on a group of individuals, by a Dr. J.C. Fahnestock (Murphy, 1995). It is not clear what dose or form of echinacea was used in the proving, or how many subjects were involved. The symptoms observed were:

accelerated pulse
biting, tingling sensation of the tongue and lips*
drowsiness*
fever
flushed face
full head*
griping pains of offensive gas*
languor*
loose yellowish bowel movements*
mucus formation in the digestive and respiratory
    tracts*
neuralgic pains*
sense of fear and pain about the heart

*Symptoms also noted in Eclectic literature or contemporary clinical studies.

Most of the symptoms are identical to those observed by the Eclectics or in contemporary German clinical studies. The fever, flushed face, and accelerated pulse noted in the provings is the opposite of the observations of the Eclectics, who noted a decreased pulse and lowered temperature with high doses of echinacea. The tendency to mucus discharge was not formally listed as a side effect by the Eclectics, but was definitely noted as a clinical effect in all their literature (Felter and Lloyd, 1898; Felter, 1922; Ellingwood, 1919). Because of this effect, homeopath William Boericke suggested in 1924 that echinacea should not be used in some cases of appendicitis; by promoting the discharge of pus, an abscessed appendix "would probably rupture sooner under its use." Boericke also lists "aching in the limbs" as a key side effect (Boericke, 1922).

Joint Pain

Ellingwood noted joint pain as a possible side effect of high doses of echinacea. I have received practitioner reports of the same symptoms with normal therapeutic doses that were taken for more than a month. Both the husband and wife who were taking echinacea noted joint pains after about a month, which went away when the physician had them stop taking the echinacea (Stansbury, 1994). To suggest more definitively that echinacea was the culprit, rather than the joint pain coming from some other unidentified cause, the patients would have had to take it again and have the joint pains return. The practitioner, who was personally skeptical that the echinacea had caused the problem, was nevertheless reluctant to prescribe it again.

In another case, presented by Samuel Masini, N.D., of Connecticut, a woman's feet actually grew a full shoe size over the course of about three weeks of taking echinacea (Masini, 1992). She was taking it in a formula in a dose of about thirty drops twice a day. This is not a large dose, but the woman was small, weighing 110 pounds. The complete formula, which was for acne, included:

Echinacea spp. (species not stated)	27 drops
Phytolacca decandra (poke root)	10 drops
Capsicum annum (cayenne pepper)	2 drops
Rumex crispus (yellow dock)	27 drops
Arctium lappa (burdock root)	27 drops
Berberis aquifolium (Oregon grape root)	27 drops

The woman took this twice a day in water or juice. Dr. Masini noted that the soft tissues of the feet were not swollen, and that the feet had grown in length rather than width. He refilled the formula without the echinacea, and the feet returned to normal in two to three days. He postulated that echinacea's ability to promote hyaluronic acid, a mucus-like gel prominent in the joints, caused the many joints in the feet to swell slightly, collectively lengthening the foot.

Neither of these cases proves that echinacea can cause joint pain, because none of the patients were "rechallenged" with the herb to see if the symptoms returned. However, the reports of joint pain are consistent with the reports of the Eclectics and the homeopaths, and it would be prudent to watch for such signs when taking echinacea over the long term. Modern research has even suggested the mechanism which might cause the pain—the "thickening" of the hyaluronic acid lubricant in the joints—as speculated by Dr. Masini. Echinacea is all too frequently promoted as being completely without side effects, so if such symptoms appear, practitioners and the public alike are unlikely to attribute the discomfort to the plant.

OTHER CAUTIONS

In Chapter 6, I described the German use of echinacea by injection. This method of administration requires specially prepared and sterilized forms of echinacea, and should not be engaged in as a home experiment with echinacea tinctures. This may seem obvious, but I receive occasional correspondence from people wondering if they can inject a tincture safely. Even if a person knows how to safely administer an injection, abscesses and serious systemic infections can result from using unpurified plant material.

Another possible complication may arise if you take echinacea before surgery—which is a good idea to prevent infection. This may raise the white blood cell count, which is a good thing, but be sure that your doctor knows you are taking echinacea and that it may have this effect. Otherwise, a doctor who performs a blood test just before surgery may conclude that an infection is causing the proliferation of white blood cells.

CONCLUSION

In normal medicinal doses, echinacea has few side effects, and the most common ones, such as belching, are minor. Side effects such as headache or joint pain may occur, especially with long-term use—more than three weeks—or with high doses. Habitually suppressing colds, flu, or other infections with echinacea may mask lifestyle causes or other illnesses, which could result in more serious or painful conditions.

To use echinacea safely, and with the least likelihood of side effects, take the following into consideration:

- Doses of less than 500 mg are least likely to cause digestive side effects. Taking echinacea before meals instead of on an empty stomach also helps.
- Don't apply echinacea tincture directly to inflamed tissues without diluting it. Take it with some warm water orally, or dilute it about 1:6 for topical use.
- If you have frequent infections or colds, don't repeatedly self-medicate with echinacea visit a practitioner of natural medicine for a checkup, including a review of your lifestyle and diet. See Chapter 10 for a description of the effects of different lifestyle factors on your immune system.

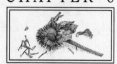

CHAPTER 8

ADULTERATION
AND
SUBSTITUTION

Adulteration of echinacea products in North America is such a potential problem that I'll describe it here in detail. The chances are good that if you've ever bought an echinacea product in North America, you've inadvertently purchased an adulterant. As we'll see below, until the last decade even physicians and scientists weren't sure what was being sold to them as "echinacea," and it remains a very real question for the public in North America today.

PARTHENIUM INTEGRIFOLIUM

In the mid-1980s, German researchers at the University of Munich apparently discovered some new constituents in *E. purpurea* (Bauer, Khan, et al, 1985). They later published an article on identification standards for *E. purpurea* and *E. angustifolia* on the basis of these constituents (Bauer, Khan, et al, 1986), and even obtained a German patent on the constituents (Wagner et al, 1987).

Later in 1986, however, the researchers discovered that the plant material supposed to be *E. purpurea* in the experiments was an entirely different plant: *Parthenium integrifolium*. They made the discovery public at a European pharmaceutical conference (Bauer, Khan, Jurcic, et al., 1986).

Parthenium has been an adulterant of commercial supplies of echinacea since at least 1909 (Moser, 1910). It does not look anything like echinacea and does not share its medicinal properties. Its root, however, when cut and sifted, looks like the much more expensive *E. angustifolia* root. Its most common name, one sometimes appearing on the labels of North American products, is Missouri snakeroot. Other names are American feverfew, cutting almond, nephritic plant, prairie dock, and wild quinine (Foster, 1991). It grows in much of the eastern U.S. Historically, it was used as a diuretic for genitourinary complaints—hence the name "nephritic plant" (nephron = part of the kidney)—and as an aromatic bitter for digestive problems. The flowering tops were once used for malaria—hence the name "wild quinine," as quinine was a common malaria medicine.

The extent of the adulteration problem has never been quantified, but in a 1987 letter to the *American Herb Association Newsletter*, the University of Munich researchers who had discovered the problem stated that all twenty commercial samples of the root they had tested were, in fact, parthenium (Bauer and Wagner, 1987). The samples had been obtained in the U.S. In the time between the publication of Bauer's original article and the discovery of the adulteration of the samples, several companies in the U.S. had their own products tested and advertised them as the "real" echinacea according to the criteria in Bauer's article. They, like Bauer, had actually obtained parthenium. Herbalist and echinacea expert Christopher Hobbs states in his 1990 book on echinacea: ". . . most of the commercially available root of *Echinacea purpurea* on the U.S. market before about 1988 was in fact *Parthenium* (Hobbs, 1990)."

This accidental discovery, like many scientific discoveries, has led to better standards of identification of echinacea plant material. Bauer and others have subsequently published detailed methods for distinguishing among the three major echinacea species and parthenium (Bauer and Wagner, 1990), and researchers and companies now have methods for detecting adulteration if they wish to do so. The discovery also cast a shadow on much of the scientific research into echinacea prior to 1989; for all studies which used plant material purchased in the U.S., there is no way now to know whether the material was echinacea or parthenium.

THE *ECHINACEA PALLIDA* PROBLEM

Steven Foster, a pioneer of echinacea research and education during the last several decades of the herbal renaissance in the U.S., has helped educate industry and herbalists in the U.S. about adulteration problems in the 1980s (Foster, 1985a, 1985b, 1987). Foster has also pointed out another problem with adulteration: the common substitution of *E. pallida* for *E. angustifolia*, which I described briefly in Chapters 1 and 2. The two species apparently were used interchangeably by the Eclectics, many of whom seem to have been ignorant of the botanical differences between them. Throughout the Eclectic medical texts, the range of *E. angustifolia* is given as eastward into Illinois. In fact, little *E. angustifolia* grows east of the

Kansas-Missouri state line, and anything found in Illinois is likely to be *E. pallida*. Native Americans apparently held that the roots of *E. pallida* were an inferior medicine to those of *E. angustifolia*. The Eclectics may have inadvertently cast their own negative vote on the quality of *E. pallida* with statements such as one by the prominent pharmacist John Uri Lloyd, who stated that echinacea grown east of the Mississippi is of a "negative quality" (Felter and Lloyd, 1898).

Because *E. angustifolia* does not grow east of the Mississippi, the variation in quality Lloyd describes was probably due to adulteration with *E. pallida*, which grows in the area and habitat he describes. Lloyd goes on to say that the best quality roots come from "the prairie lands of Nebraska," the natural habitat for *E. angustifolia*, but not of the other species (Felter and Lloyd, 1898). Foster says that such adulteration is still a major problem in the U.S. echinacea supply, although that problem, like adulteration with parthenium, has never been quantified (Foster, 1991).

The discovery of adulteration of *E. angustifolia* with *E. pallida*, like the adulteration with parthenium, has also cast doubt on research into *E. angustifolia* prior to the late 1980s. There is now no way to know whether research supposed to be on *E. angustifolia* was actually done on *E. pallida* samples before that time, when careful identification of plant material became routine.

LET THE BUYER BEWARE

In the late 1980s, when the scandal of echinacea adulteration spread in the herbal world, some companies moved to ensure that they had properly identified their product. Parthenium is less expensive than echinacea, and some companies have ignored the problem. At least some of what is sold in the U.S. as echinacea is undoubtedly parthenium. The way I handle the problem, personally, is to buy products only from companies that carefully identify or grow their own echinacea. A list of some of my favorites is found in Appendix B.

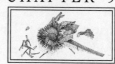

CHAPTER 9

IS ONE SPECIES "BEST"?

Echinacea was resurrected as a popular herb in the U.S. in the late 1970s and early 1980s. Since that time, herbalists and the general public have been debating whether one species is better than the other as a medicine. In the following section, I'll review the arguments for the different species, give you my own opinion, and then let you decide for yourself. I invite you to buy (or even better, grow) some of each, try them out, and be the judge yourself.

NATIVE AMERICAN AND EARLY COLONIAL USE

We have very little knowledge of Native American use of *E. purpurea* (see Table 2.1). This could be because the Native Americans did not use it as a medicine, or because ethnobotanical information was not collected before the eastern tribes that may have used it were resettled on western reservations. The native uses of *E. angustifolia* and *E. pallida* were apparently quite extensive, although use was most widespread in territories in which *E. angustifolia* is native (Bauer and Wagner, 1991). It was the Native use of *E. angustifolia* that brought echinacea into general medical practice in the U.S., first through its introduction into the literature by Rafinesque, and then through the work of Meyer, King, and Lloyd. Thus, ethnobotanical studies would support *E. angustifolia* as the most important species.

The early colonists apparently used *E. purpurea* in veterinary medicine. There is also occasional mention of its use as a "household medicine" for digestive complaints, and mention of it as a treatment for venereal disease (Foster, 1991). There is no mention of its ability to heal the wide variety of conditions for which we find *E. angustifolia* useful, however. You have to ask, if the *E. purpurea* root is equivalent to *E. angustifolia*, and if it was in use by the colonists and Native Americans of the eastern U.S. for such things as indigestion, how did its other remarkable healing properties escape their notice for so many centuries? Why did the non-Native-American world have to wait until 1885, when *E. angustifolia* was introduced into medical practice, to discover the immune-system-stimulating properties of this remarkable plant?

THE ECLECTICS

The Eclectic physicians held unequivocally that the *E. angustifolia* species was the best. The only mention of *E. purpurea* in their early literature (pre-1886) was for veterinary uses (Rafinesque, 1830). There are a few mentions made of *E. purpurea* in Eclectic literature in the last decade of the 1800s (Felter and Lloyd, 1898; Cook, 1892), but by the 1920s, it had been dropped completely by the Eclectics as a medicine (Felter, 1922; Ellingwood, 1919). In 1898, Felter mentions *E. purpurea* as a plant worthy of further investigation (Felter and Lloyd, 1898), but by 1922 he omits any mention of it at all (Felter, 1922). Professor Ellingwood wrote in 1919:

> *There is considerable confusion concerning the iden-tity of the active medicinal species of echinacea. The E. purpurea of the Eastern States has been thought to be identical with the E. angustifolia of the Western States. It is often used for the same purposes, but is universally disappointing.*

> (Ellingwood, 1919)

Even the Eclectic giant and echinacea expert, John Uri Lloyd, wrote:

> *Much of the root collected has little medicinal value. This is due not to poorly kept and cured roots alone, but chiefly to the locality in which it grows. Much of the drug collected in the marshes and lowlands east of the Mississippi is of this negative quality.*

> (Felter and Lloyd, 1898)

Here Lloyd is referring to the region and natural habi-tat of *E. pallida* and *E. purpurea*. The purpurea species can grow in moist areas better than the other two species can. Lloyd also states (Lloyd, 1897): "The best quality root comes from the prairie lands of Nebraska"—the area in which *E. angustifolia* is native.

GERMAN EXPERIENCE

The preceding information would seem to make an unequivocal case for *E. angustifolia* as the better medicinal species, but we have more facts to consider. We saw in Chapter 1 that *E. purpurea* entered into medical use in the 1930s as the result of a mistake, when Dr. Madaus of Germany purchased *E. purpurea* seeds that were mislabeled as *E. angustifolia*. German homeopaths had already introduced the widespread use of *E. angustifolia* there. Subsequent German experience with *E. purpurea* flowering tops has shown it to be an effective clinical medicine, whether in oral, topical, or injectable forms. Research in petri dishes and animals even suggests that *E. purpurea* constituents are more potent than those in *E. angustifolia*. Clinical research into a tincture of the *E. purpurea* root showed it to be an effective medicine, in high doses, for flu-like cold symptoms. In short, German experience and research proves that *E. purpurea* is not, as Ellingwood stated, "universally disappointing."

There is, however, no consensus in Germany that *E. purpurea* is in any way superior to *E. angustifolia*. Although some writers state that *E. purpurea* is the most popular species there, as measured by sales volume (Beuscher et al, 1995), there are many more *E. angustifolia* products in the German marketplace. In their 1990 German-language echinacea handbook, researchers Bauer and Wagner list 229 commercial products (sixty-six of them in homeopathic dilutions) in Germany containing *E. angustifolia,* and only seventy-two containing *E. purpurea* (nine homeopathic dilutions).

RECONCILING THE FACTS

How purpurea could have been experimented with and rejected so soundly by the Eclectics, then later used with success by the Germans, is a mystery that has not been solved. But as powerful as such testimony by the Eclectics may seem, there are several reasons why they could have been mistaken about the powers of *E. purpurea*.

First, we saw in Chapter 1 that echinacea supplies have been adulterated with look-alike roots such as *Parthenium integrifolium* and other herbs from the time of the Eclectics right up until today. According to Foster (1991), there has never been a significant amount of wild *E. purpurea* in the marketplace. It only became common in the U.S. in the last decade when it has been cultivated in large quantities. Thus it is possible that, in the time of the Eclectics, when *E. purpurea* was not cultivated, whatever was sold as *E. purpurea* was more likely to be a worthless adulterant, thus ruining the reputation of the plant.

Another possibility is that the Eclectics judged the quality of echinacea not by clinical observation, but by the tingling sensation the root induces on the tongue. We saw in Chapter 5 that *E. angustifolia* has more of the tingle-producing isobutylamides than does *E. purpurea*. Other less-tasty constituents in *E. purpurea* could also contribute to immune-system-stimulating activity, but leave a less dramatic impression on the herbalist judging the quality.

CONTEMPORARY OPINION

I am primarily an herbal clinician and educator. I use herbs as medicines, and I don't know a lot about growing them or harvesting them in the wild. Although my initial training was as a scientist, and I have nothing against science, for my purposes as a clinician, I will always prefer the report of an experienced physician or herbalist working with real patients to that of a scientist working with animals or cell cultures in a petri dish—a scientist who may never have given a medicine to a patient or conducted a careful interview to assess the results.

In my role as an educator and as editor of *Medical Herbalism*, a clinical newsletter, I come in contact with many practicing physicians and herbalists in North America. I have observed that *E. angustifolia* was considered more potent clinically until the 1990s, when reliable sources of unadulterated *E. purpurea* became available. Since that time, practitioners seem to feel that the two species are interchangeable; if one is not working, then you need a different herb, not the other species.

While writing this book, I have informally interviewed many of these herbalists to get their private opinions on the matter of which species is best, and I put the question to a group of professional herbalists on the Internet. The verdict is a complete toss-up. I found no one who stated that one species was unequivocally better than the other, and about half the practitioners held each of the species as a personal favorite. A good reason to prefer the purpurea species is that what is available in the marketplace is invariably cultivated instead of harvested in the wild. This allows for more accurate plant identification, lessens the likelihood of adulteration, and reduces the strain on endangered plant populations in the wild. My own personal preference is for *E. angustifolia* because I like the more potent tingling sensation that it produces.

CHAPTER 10

CAUSES OF IMMUNE SYSTEM WEAKNESS

In Chapter 11, I will describe how to take echinacea for infections and chronic immune system weakness. In following chapters, I'll describe a number of other useful herbs. But before I do so, I will describe here the causes of immune system weakness.

In my clinical work, I think in terms of a healing "triangle":

1. lifestyle and diet
2. spiritual vitality
3. herbal treatment

Immune system weakness invariably arises from the first two areas, not from an "herb deficiency." If you eat a diet rich in heavy, poor-quality, or incompatible foods; suffer from chronic stress; take drugs for every ache, pain, and discomfort;

indulge in addictions to destructive substances; feel a lack of connectedness to life and nature; take a self-centered approach to your fellows; feel no sense of creativity and purpose in life; and hold no feeling of the sacredness of the Creator and creation, it would be foolhardy to expect echinacea or any other herb to make up for these irregularities. It is wiser and saner to view herbs as allies—as helping gifts of nature—while you seek to grow in your understanding and mastery of your life and health.

SUGAR

Americans consume about five ounces of sugar every day, either consciously added to their food or hidden in the processed foods they eat. That's more than a quarter of a pound. Scientific studies have found that amounts lower than this can profoundly suppress the immune system. In one study, three ounces of sucrose at one sitting reduced the ability of phagocytes to engulf bacteria and other invaders by about forty percent. The effect started within half an hour and last more than five hours (Sanchez et al, 1973; Ringsdorf et al, 1976). Another trial showed that only two ounces of glucose suppressed the activity of B- and T-lymphocytes (Bernstein, 1977). This applies to sugars that naturally occur in food as well.

This doesn't mean that you can't eat apples, oranges, or carrots, which are all sweet by nature. But do use caution with frequent high doses of concentrates of these, such as fruit juices. While large doses of concentrated juices may contain high amounts of vitamins and minerals, they also contain sugars in the immuno-suppressive range. Some individuals, while fasting, make the mistake of drinking sugary fruit juices instead of the milder vegetable juices, thereby losing some of the benefits of the fast by inhibiting their immune systems.

If a company were to introduce sugar for the first time as a food additive today, under current FDA guidelines, they would be laughed out of the department. Only because it was in traditional use when the department was formed is it currently allowed to be added to foods — and it is added to everything from catsup, to bread, to fast-food french fries. Box 10.1 shows some of the names for sugar that you will find on product labels. A typical sugared soft drink or serving of ice-cream contains enough sugar to depress your immune system. Sugar consumption in North America is a major cause of immune system weakness. I tell my patients to go ahead and feast on something sweet one or two days a week if they want to, but to eliminate the habit of eating sweets daily.

FOOD ALLERGIES

Many North Americans have hidden food allergies that deplete their immune systems. If the food is eaten habitually, as allergenic foods often are, a huge amount of antigenic material must be handled, exhausting resources that could be allocated to invading microorganisms or cancer cells. If you have an allergy to dairy products, the body treats that quarter pound of cheese and two glasses of milk a day just the same as if it were a quarter pound of bacteria and three glasses of a virus. The resulting exhaustion of the immune system impairs the body's ability to respond to other threats.

Researchers have found that white blood cell counts can drop by as much as fifty percent after a single serving of allergenic food (Rinkel et al, 1951). The cells don't just

BOX 10.1

HIDDEN SUGAR IN YOUR FOOD

Following are some of the names for
sugars that may appear on the labels of
processed foods. All are immunosuppressive
in the amounts consumed by the average
American.

barley malt	invert sugar
beet sugar	lactose
brown sugar	levulose
cane sugar	maltose
corn syrup	milk sugar
date sugar	rice syrup
dextrose	succinate
fructose	sucrose
high-fructose corn syrup	turbinado sugar
honey	

disappear, however. They migrate to the scene of the allergen invasion: the lymphatics in the throat and intestines. These nodes become engorged, and the bacteria that they would otherwise eliminate can proliferate there. The "infection" will invariably be blamed on the germs, but the underlying cause is the food allergen overload. Food allergies can thus play a predominant role in sore throats, tonsillitis, upper respiratory infections, and childhood ear infections. In one clinical trial, 104 children with ear "infections" were screened for food allergies. Eighty-one had allergies to such foods as dairy products and wheat, the most common allergenic foods. The ear problems improved when the foods were removed from the diet and returned when the foods were reintroduced (Pennisi, 1994).

If you have a weak immune system, one clue that you may have a food allergy is a craving for a particular food or foods. A day or even a meal would not be complete without that food. This type of food "addiction" is a common sign of food allergy. Try eliminating the food completely for six weeks (it won't be easy), weathering the withdrawal symptoms. Then reintroduce it and see what symptoms reappear. You might also consult with a practitioner of natural medicine about screening for food allergies. The most common allergies are to dairy products and wheat.

Elimination of food allergens, along with elimination of sugar, is the most common intervention I suggest to immune-system-deficient patients at my clinic.

ALCOHOL

Moderate amounts of alcohol probably have no serious effect on immunity. Amounts sufficient to cause intoxication, however, can profoundly suppress the immune system. Statistics show that infectious diseases—especially pneumonia—are much more common among habitual drinkers (Baker and Jerrells, 1993).

A study of more than 1,100 undergraduate students at a midwestern university found that students drinking an average of more than twenty-two drinks per week had significantly more upper respiratory infections and acute illnesses than did students who drank less than that. Students consuming more than twenty-eight drinks had significantly more illnesses of all types (Engs and Aldo-Benson, 1995).

Whether consumed habitually, or only occasionally in amounts sufficient to cause intoxication, alcohol has adverse effects on all major components of the immune system. It affects the levels of both phagocytes and lymphocytes and depresses their activity. The effects last for about two weeks after stopping habitual drinking and do not return to normal for two months or more (Mili et al., 1992; Tonnesen et al., 1992).

NUTRITIONAL DEFICIENCIES

Nutritional deficiencies, especially those associated with immune system deficiency, are common in the U.S. Every survey appearing in the literature on the nutritional status of Americans in the last thirty years has found that not everyone was getting all their nutrients at the level of recommended dietary allowances. Natural physicians consider even these recommended levels as too low to maintain optimum immunity. Deficiencies of vitamins A, B12, C, folic acid, pantothenic acid, pyridoxine, riboflavin, copper, and zinc have been associated with immune system deficiency. Table 10.1 shows the frequency of deficiencies of these vitamins and minerals in the U.S. population.

PESTICIDES

Pesticides can put a strain on the immune system, robbing it of resources that it needs to fight its natural enemies. They

TABLE 10.1   DEFICIENCIES OF VITAMINS
AND MINERALS ASSOCIATED
WITH IMMUNE SYSTEM STATUS
IN THE U.S. POPULATION

Vitamin A	Occasionally deficient in the elderly.
Vitamin B12	Often deficient in the elderly.
Vitamin C	20–40% of U.S. women have Vitamin C intake below 42 mg. The current RDA is 200 mg. The actual need for optimum immunity may be 1–3 grams/day. Other risk groups: men who live alone; those who avoid acid-containing foods such as oranges because of heartburn or sensitivity; alcoholics; smokers.
Copper	Two clinical reviews found that 75–81% of the American population fails to consume the RDA of copper in their diets.
Folic acid	Often deficient in the elderly, from 22%–100% in surveys of various elderly populations.
Pyridoxine	Often deficient in the elderly despite "adequate" dietary intake (30%–83% are deficient). 50% of pregnant women are deficient.
Riboflavin	Often deficient in the elderly (10–30% are deficient). 26% of the impoverished are deficient.
Zinc	Low in 87% of elderly. 68% of Americans consume less than two-thirds of the RDA. Usually deficient in children and teenagers. Pregnant women consume only about two-thirds of their requirements.

(Source: Werbach, 1987)

are potent immune system suppressors, having an adverse
effect on the T- and B-cells of the specific immune system defenses (Rae and Liang, 1991). They are now ubiquitous in
the environment, especially in the food we eat.

My Experience with Pesticides

In the early 1980s, I ran a large natural food store in New Haven, Connecticut, that specialized in high-quality produce, although most of it was not organic. Each morning I would go to the produce terminal before dawn, poke through eighty to one hundred different boxes of produce, and pick the highest grade and quality available for our department. In the course of doing so, I was exposed to whatever pesticides were on the produce, which could have been a dozen or more, including banned pesticides such as DDT.

One time, several of my employees complained about having to package some spinach, saying that it was causing a rash on their hands. I was skeptical, thinking they were trying to get out of the work, but I let them do something else and began to package it myself. Within sixty seconds, a rash had spread from my wrists to my elbows and was moving up my arm. I later asked the owner of the produce company where I got the spinach what might be on it. He averted his eyes, acted evasive, and said "Well, you never know what's on the stuff." That same year, three brothers in one family—all owners of one of the produce houses in the terminal who had handled pesticide-laden produce since childhood—all died of cancer.

Before and after this time in my adult life, I've had an unusually strong immune system, only getting a cold or flu every three or four years. But after about three years of this regular exposure to pesticides, I developed severe chronic fatigue. I was so exhausted that my doctor told me to go to bed for two weeks. I was only slightly better after that. During this time I also developed multiple allergies to foods. I had no clue that pesticides were the problem, but I gradually recovered when I delegated that work to someone else, and eventually left the produce trade completely. Only in retrospect did it occur to me that the pesticides on the produce were the problem. Despite a battery of medical tests by both conventional and alternative physicians, no one ever found the cause of my condition.

This is more than just a personal anecdote. The pesticide combinations I was exposed to were identical to the ones you eat on commercial produce every day. My exposure may have been more intense, but pesticides are likely to have at least some effect on your immune system.

A Case Study

I am currently treating a patient in his mid-thirties who is built like a horse, exercises regularly, and has a good diet. But he has a serious immune system deficiency, causing frequent colds and infections, night sweats, and general malaise. His profession: He is a horticulturist who works in a greenhouse and on a farm growing roses. Three days a week, his job is to "fog" the greenhouse with pesticides and other chemicals. Even though he wears a mask and a protective suit when he does so, for the rest of the week he works eight to twelve hours a day in this pesticide-drenched environment. I have had no success in restoring his health, even with the full armament of immune-system-stimulating herbs. He will have to change his profession before he will recover.

Reducing Exposure

You can reduce pesticide levels in your diet by seeking out organic produce, or by washing and scrubbing your commercial produce thoroughly. Range-fed meats, which are available in most larger health food stores, are also advisable. Pesticides tend to accumulate as you move higher up the food chain; an ear of corn may have only low levels of pesticide residues, but bushels of that corn fed to a pig or other animal may cause much larger amounts of the pesticide to accumulate in the animal's fat. If you eat meat from the animal, you get more pesticides than you could ever accumulate by eating corn.

More significant than dietary pesticides are those you are exposed to in the workplace, or even in your own front yard. In Colorado, where I live, more pesticides are used on lawns in the cities than in all the agriculture in the state combined.

Pharmaceutical Drugs

The chronic use of many drugs depresses the immune system, including those drugs most often given for infections and inflammation.

Antibiotics

The most serious culprits are antibiotic drugs taken for long periods. A short course of antibiotics is appropriate for serious infections. Unfortunately, antibiotics are often prescribed inappropriately for the common cold and flu and other conditions for which science shows they are ineffective. They are also prescribed for months or years for such conditions as acne.

Short-term antibiotic use can cause unpleasant side effects, but long-term use can be devastating to the immune system. The antibiotics disrupt the healthy bacteria in the gut, which normally hold disease-causing bacteria and yeast in check. The bowel then can become toxic, poisoning the system from within. Candida yeast can overgrow in the intestine, and vaginal yeast infections may also arise. The intestinal yeast infection can then cause lesions in the intestinal wall, resulting in a syndrome known as "leaky gut." Large food molecules and intestinal bacteria can then cross the intestine wall, creating a tremendous overload on the immune system. Multiple food allergies can result. This syndrome, in its worst stages, is absolutely devastating.

We have a patient at our clinic who was unable to work for a year, spent most of her day in bed, had lost twenty pounds, and could only eat eight foods without an allergic reaction. Previously, she had taken antibiotics and steroid drugs almost continuously for about a decade. We are gradually restoring her health by restoring the health of her digestive tract.

Pain Medications and Steroids

Pain medications are sold by the hundred of tons each year in the U.S. The daily per capita consumption of aspirin alone is about two tablets a day. Pain medications work by turning off the inflammatory response. See Box 4.1 for a list of the healthy effects of the inflammatory reaction. While they may reduce the immediate pain, these drugs also depress the immune system.

In a clinical trial, patients who were experimentally infected with a virus that causes the common cold were given various pain medications or a placebo. Those taking aspirin and acetaminophen had worse symptoms and a lowered production of antibodies than those taking the placebo (Graham,

1990). Steroid drugs, such as are commonly used to suppress allergies, asthma, and skin conditions, are even more suppressive, decreasing the number of white blood cells, the activity of phagocytes, the movement of immune system cells to the site of infection, and the production of interferon (Dale and Federman, 1995). Pain medications and steroids can also, like the antibiotics, cause the "leaky gut" syndrome.

So important is the effect of such immune system suppression by drugs that I consider it impossible for my chronic disease patients to recover if they are using them habitually in any dosage.

STRESS

Stress is a natural part of life. When faced with a life-threatening situation, the body's sympathetic nervous system becomes predominant. This hastens the release of energy, increases blood flow to the muscles, and prepares the body for a short period of extreme exertion. This "fight-or-flight" response, if severe enough, enables a person under stress to perform superhuman acts, like lifting a car off an injured person or heroically saving the lives of fellow soldiers. This response also temporarily depresses the immune system.

Less serious situations, such as an important crisis on the job, an impending deadline, or urgent needs of children in the home, also involve this sympathetic nervous system response. Under ideal conditions, such situations are rare, and when the danger has passed, the body can return to a more normal state. When resting, relaxing, eating, or sleeping, the parasympathetic nervous system is predominant. During this phase, the body builds and repairs and stores up energy for future use, and the immune system does most of its work.

Unfortunately, many of us remain locked in the "sympathetic" state as we meet the complexity of modern civilization. Our hunter-gatherer and agrarian ancestors only faced life-threatening stress occasionally, during hunting or warfare, and spent much of their time relaxing. Anthropologists say that our hunter-gatherer predecessors worked a three-day week and spent the rest of their time in sport, recreation, music, dancing, family life, or ritual. Many of us today relax only rarely, working more than forty hours a week in high-stress jobs or family situations. We don't relax or enjoy exercise enough, or our relaxation is of poor quality, such as watching television. The result is exhaustion, indigestion, insomnia, depletion of the immune system, chronic illness, and other ill effects of a prolonged sympathetic state. The remedy, of course, is stress management and improved quality and quantity of rest and relaxation. Tonic herbs and foods are also appropriate for this condition, and for any condition accompanied by depleted energy.

The Pathology of Stress

Chronic low-grade stress, without proper rest and recuperation in the parasympathetic state, can have devastating effects on the immune system. The chief culprit is the hormone *cortisol*, which is secreted by the adrenal gland. Normally the body reduces the production of cortisol after a short period, through a feedback loop to the *hypothalamus* in the brain. Then, during sleep, other secretions of the adrenals called *androgens*—including the DHEA so popular in health food stores today—become predominant. The adrenal androgens aid in restoration and repair of the body.

With chronic stress, the feedback loop to the hypothalamus loses its efficiency, and chronically elevated cortisol levels result. Insomnia is often the first noticeable symptom. Cortisol is an immune system suppressant, just like the pharmaceutical corticosteroids, but about one-fourth as strong. It suppresses all levels of the immune system, and especially the all-important T-helper cells. With cortisol-induced sleep disturbances, the cortisol continues to depress the immune system during the night hours, when it customarily does its best work. The restorative effects of the androgens is also diminished, and immune system deficiency and degenerative diseases result. Thus "stress" is a contributor to colds, flu, and other infections, and rest and recuperation is essential to healthy recovery.

Sleep Deprivation

We know from pioneer diaries that, in the last century, Americans slept about nine hours a night. Scientific studies show that if you let people sleep until they wake up, they will sleep about eight-and-a-half hours. In 1970, Americans slept an average of seven-and-a-half hours a night, and by 1990 they slept for only seven hours, on average. A third of us sleep less than six hours a night. The immune system does its work when we are resting or at night when we are asleep.

These sleep levels create a chronic, slow drain on immunity. In one clinical trial, a group of men were deprived of four hours of sleep for one night. Their natural killer cell level—our most important weapon against virus infection and cancer—had fallen by nearly a third the next day (Anon., 1995).

In my clinical work, I often adopt an initial strategy of restoring sleep for patients with chronic illnesses who also suffer from insomnia or stress, using such herbs as skullcap, passionflower, valerian, lemon balm, and kava-kava. This allows the body to perform its normal immunity and restoration functions, and reduces the need for more heroic treatments of the chronic symptoms.

Exercise-Induced Stress

Excessive exercise is one form of stress. Sufficient exercise is absolutely necessary for the functioning of the immune system. The muscular movements promote the healthy flow of lymph, and the pumping of the diaphragm promotes the detoxifying actions of the liver and spleen. But overdoing it, especially habitually, can depress your immune system.

Exercising to the point of pain or exhaustion depresses the immune system for several hours after stopping. Habitually exercising to this point two or more times a week increases the likelihood of infection (Baenkler, 1992). Studies of people who train for and race in marathons show a dramatic depression of immunity. In one study, racers who finished a marathon were six times more likely to get a cold or flu after the race than were runners who registered but did not run (Eichner, 1993).

I see this problem in our clinic most often in women who overexercise to control their weight. This is part of the pattern of anorexia and bulimia; obsession with the figure results in irrational behavior to control it. A recent patient, for instance, was exhausted and depleted, with poor digestion and many manifestations of immune system weakness. She was also underweight, with a history of anorexia. In spite of this, she exercised for about an hour most days. In doing so, she was exhausting her immune system as well as her adrenal glands. On my advice, as part of a larger overall program, she reduced this exercise to thirty minutes three or four times a week, and continued daily relaxing walks rather than heavy jogging. Along with other treatments and lifestyle changes she is gradually recovering. This is the level of exercise I recommend for most people: aerobic exercise, but not to the point of pain or exhaustion, three times a week, and gentler exercise, like walking, for half an hour every day.

SPIRITUAL CONSIDERATIONS

The writer who has influenced me the most in my studies of natural healing is Dr. Henry Lindlahr, a founder of the modern naturopathic medical profession who ran a 200-bed inpatient facility in Chicago in the early decades of this century. He became a physician in his forties, and treated more than twenty-five thousand patients before his death, using methods such as hydrotherapy, diet, spinal manipulation, and homeopathy, with remarkable success on the full range of human disease. Although licensed as an M.D., he wrote no more than fifty drug prescriptions in his entire career. He was so in demand that waiting lists for entry into his establishment were common. Patients included a large number of individuals considered terminally insane, with whom he claimed a fifty-percent cure rate. He encouraged his patients, in a non-denominational and non-dogmatic way, to undertake daily prayer and positive mental affirmations, and considered these to be indispensable in treating the psychological component of chronic disease.

A large body of scientific literature now exists showing a connection between your thoughts, attitudes, and emotions and the state of your immune system. A detailed review is beyond the scope of this book. One strong indication in this literature is a connection between prayer—either praying or being prayed for—and health. Various studies show that overall health, mental health, freedom from addictions, and immune system status are benefited by prayer, regardless of religious denomination. For a general review of the literature, see Davis (1994).

Daily prayer and group prayer reduce stress and depression, presumably with a positive effect on the immune system (see the section on stress and immunity above). One study showed improved immune system status in AIDS patients who prayed or meditated regularly (Carson, 1993). A well-designed double-blind controlled trial showed that being prayed *for* improved the status of heart-attack patients in an acute coronary care center (Byrd, 1988). Prayer is also considered an essential element in recovery from addictions, and provides assistance and a positive attitude toward lifestyle improvements in general.

If prayer, meditation, and a spiritual approach to life can help patients with such serious immune system disorders as AIDS, or such devastating physical conditions as heart attacks, they certainly have a place in less serious conditions. I, like Dr. Lindlahr, consider them essential to the cure of chronic illness and the attainment of optimal health. I encourage my patients to find a religion or other path that is compatible with them, and to engage in prayer or meditation as a daily habit.

CONCLUSION

In the remaining chapters of the book, I will tell you how to use echinacea and a number of other herbs to treat colds, flu, infections, and chronic immune system weakness. I would encourage you, if you have chronic immune system weakness, to study this chapter and identify as many of the causes of your condition as possible. Removing these causes will make the greatest contribution to your recovery.

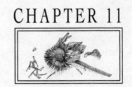

CHAPTER 11

How to Use Echinacea

In this chapter, I will describe the products available today in health food stores, including a few brand names. I'll tell you how to make your own echinacea products. And I'll tell you how to use echinacea. I advise you to review Chapters 7 and 10 before using echinacea for periods of more than a month.

Product Types

You may find many different forms of echinacea in the health food store or herb shop. Each may have advantages or disadvantages, which I will describe below.

Whole Roots

Whole echinacea roots are available in many health food stores today. This is one of the best ways to ensure that you are getting an unadulterated product. You can use the whole roots to make your own products, as I will describe below. Don't use whole roots to make tea, which wastes the most important active ingredients.

Tinctures

A tincture is an extraction of a plant in a mixture of alcohol and water. It will contain the alcohol-soluble products—the most important echinacea constituents—and some of the water-soluble active ingredients. If you are taking large doses of echinacea, or taking it for a long time, I suggest that you make your own tincture, as described below, and save money.

Fluid Extracts

Today you are more likely to find a fluid extract than a simple tincture of echinacea in the health food store. The tincture uses one part of plant to five parts of the water-alcohol solvent. The fluid extract typically uses one part of plant for each part of the solvent, and is thus two-and-a-half times stronger. Some fluid extracts are "vacuum concentrated" and are even more potent. The fluid extract is usually your best buy, because you can use lower doses.

Teas

Echinacea teas are almost worthless as a medicine. They do not contain the valuable alcohol-soluble constituents, and have never been used either in traditional or medical use.

Capsules and Tablets

Capsules and tablets present an advantage for people who want to avoid alcohol for reasons of taste, health, or sobriety. Two kinds of encapsulated echinacea appear in the marketplace today: powders and dehydrated extracts. The dehydrated extracts are generally more potent. If you use these products, break them open or crush them and take them in some warm water. As we saw in Chapter 6, it may be important to expose the echinacea to the lymphatics in the mouth, or to make the constituents easily absorbable in the stomach.

Freeze-Dried Products

A freeze-dried form of echinacea appeared in the marketplace in the mid-1980s. Freeze-drying herbs is a common method of standardizing plant material in laboratory or clinical trials to ensure uniformity. It is a poor concept for commercial products, however, because freeze-dried materials must be vacuum-packed and kept away from light to avoid degradation. These products have a short shelf-life and are not reliable for medical use.

Herbal Combinations

Many products exist that combine echinacea with other herbs. Some of these are well-formulated, but others contain so little echinacea that it will be of little benefit. Combinations of echinacea and goldenseal are common, but, as we will see in the following chapters, are ill-conceived. Look ahead to Box 12.3 and notice that, in the history of medical use, goldenseal has *never* been used to treat colds or flu—the most common reason why people buy these combinations today. I suggest that you learn the use of the herbs in this book, buy separate tinctures, and make your own combinations. I will describe how to do so below and in Chapter 20.

Many products combine the angustifolia and purpurea species of echinacea, and these may be superior to either tincture alone, because each has some unique immune-system-stimulating components.

Salves and Ointments

Echinacea salves and ointments are common products in Europe, useful as antiseptics and as treatments for skin ailments. Similar products have begun to appear in some health food stores. I'll describe how to make your own products for topical applications.

BRAND NAMES

The companies listed in Appendix B all make good-quality, reliable echinacea products from well-identified plant material. It's beyond the scope of this book to go into the many products in detail, but I will mention a few.

Echinagard

We saw in Chapter 6 that much of the German clinical research has been performed on a German product called Echinacin. This is a reliable product made from properly identified plant material, widely used by physicians in Europe. The same product is sold in this country, under the brand name Echinagard, by the Nature's Way company. Both liquid and capsule forms are available.

Polysaccharide-Enhanced Echinacea

Southwest herbalist Michael Moore has developed a method of extracting and preserving both the alcohol- and water-soluble constituents of echinacea. You can read about the method in his book, *Medicinal Plants of the Desert and Canyon West* (Moore, 1989). It is quite complicated to use this method, however, requiring special equipment. A number of Southwest herbalists make this extract for personal or professional use. It is also available for sale from Dancing Willow Herbs in Durango, Colorado. In a poll of professional herbalists on the Internet, this extract won a few mentions as the best form of echinacea.

MAKING YOUR OWN ECHINACEA PRODUCTS

You can easily save money by purchasing whole echinacea roots and making your own tinctures or capsules. With a little more effort, you can grow your own echinacea; *E. purpurea* grows well in a variety of climates. Seed sources are listed in Appendix B. Clip the tops about eight inches above the ground when the plant is in flower to make a juice. Harvest the roots in fall when the tops have died back, around the time of the first freeze.

Tincture

See Appendix A for directions on how to make your own echinacea tinctures.

Powder

You can purchase roots, or else dry your homegrown ones, to make powder for capsules or to add to warm water. You will have to experiment with homegrown roots and your equipment to see when they are dry enough to make a powder. Grind what you need for a few days or a week in a coffee grinder.

DOSAGE

A standard dose of echinacea when you are sick is a dropperful of tincture every two or three hours. You can use a little less of a concentrated fluid extract, or use doses of 500 milligrams of the powder. For prevention, a dropperful of tincture three times a day will suffice. At the onset of the signs of a cold or flu, take a teaspoonful every two hours. This will usually knock out the cold. If you still have the cold after four or five doses, cut back to the standard dose. We saw in Chapter 3 that the Eclectics used such a dose to cure many serious illnesses. If you have a true emergency, such as a rattlesnake bite, you can take up to half an ounce every hour while waiting for proper medical care. Use the same dose for any life-threatening infection if you are beyond the reach of medical help.

Duration

You can take echinacea for as long as you want, for instance throughout the winter or through a long flu season if you are susceptible to colds and flu. The myth that echinacea loses its immune-system-stimulating effects over time is thoroughly reviewed in Chapter 7. Look through the same chapter for a description of possible side effects from long-term use. If you are thinking of taking echinacea long term, please also reread Chapter 10 on lifestyle factors that depress the immune system function.

APPLICATIONS

Here are some ways to take or apply echinacea:

- Review Table 3.2 to see how the Eclectics used it internally and externally.
- If you take the tincture, put the drops in a small amount of warm water to reduce possible irritation of the tissues.
- Put a daily dose in a half-gallon container of water, and drink it throughout the day. Add some licorice, peppermint, or other tea for flavor if you like. This helps you maintain frequent doses, and also helps make sure you are drinking enough water.
- If you take capsules or tablets, break them open or crush them and take them with some warm water.
- For a topical wash, mix the tincture in three parts water, and apply with gauze pads. Reapply every two hours.
- To make a poultice, dilute echinacea tincture with one part water and mix with bentonite clay (available at most health food stores). Mix until the paste is just thick enough that it will not ooze. Apply the clay poultice to the skin. Change at least three times a day.

Dr. Sharol Tilgner, a naturopathic physician from Oregon, relates a case using a clay poultice for a brown recluse spider bite. A man was bitten on his thigh, and had received a prescription of antibiotics which had no effect. This type of spider puts out a poison that eats the tissues. The lesion can grow to the size of a small hand. His M.D. had advised him that if it got too bad, he would cut the tissue away. Tilgner applied the clay and gave him some to take with him. By the next day, the lesion was receding, and it eventually healed without a scar.

MAKE YOUR OWN FORMULAS

Much of the German clinical research has been into combination products, which include other plants with demonstrated immune-system-stimulating properties. Such combinations are often markedly more effective than echinacea alone. I describe a number of herbs that make good combinations with echinacea in Chapters 17 and 19. Some of the best are boneset, osha, red root, usnea, and uva ursi.

You can also boost the effects of your echinacea by adding one-tenth part of a circulatory stimulant. We saw in Chapter 3 that the Eclectics used echinacea to treat fevers; it is considered a "cooling" herb. During fever, the pulse is elevated, and the echinacea is rapidly circulated throughout the body. However, I have observed that patients without a fever—who feel cold, have a normal or low temperature, and have pale skin and a slow pulse—do not benefit from echinacea as greatly as do those with a hotter disposition or condition. The best way to overcome this problem is to add a circulatory stimulant to the echinacea. My favorites for such a combination are prickly ash bark and cayenne.

COMBINING ECHINACEA WITH
CONVENTIONAL MEDICATIONS

We saw in Chapter 6 that German researchers used echinacea along with a conventional antifungal cream to treat
vaginal yeast infections. The group receiving echinacea had
dramatically fewer recurrences. There is no reason why you
can't take echinacea along with conventional antibiotic, antifungal, or antiparasitic drugs, if you must take them. By
adding strength to the immune system, you will help the
drugs do their job more effectively. The development of resistant strains of bacteria or candida yeast overgrowth will
be less likely.

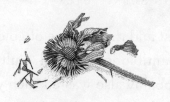

GOLDENSEAL AND ITS SUBSTITUTES

Goldenseal is the King and Queen of herbs that the Good Lord put in the ground.

A.L. Tommie Bass, traditional Appalachian herbalist

GOLDENSEAL is one of the most famous of the North American herbs. It was in use as a medicine among the eastern Native Americans when French and English colonists first arrived here and has been in continuous use ever since in both folk healing and professional medicine. Goldenseal earned its early reputation as a bitter tonic for a deranged digestive system and an antiseptic for inflammations and poorly healing wounds. Today it has a reputation as an herbal antibiotic—a reputation that I will challenge in this section—which

contributes to the high cost and the overuse of goldenseal by our germ-and-antibiotic-obsessed culture.
Tons of goldenseal are probably also wasted each year
by individuals trying to mask drug use in urine tests—
something goldenseal will not do. In this section, I will
review the history of goldenseal as a medicine, describe scientific research into its constituents, tell you
how to use it, and describe some less expensive and
more appropriate substitutes.

CHAPTER 12

GOLDENSEAL IN HISTORY

NATIVE AMERICAN USES OF GOLDENSEAL

The biography of a medicine is as interesting as that of a man.

Dr. Edwin M. Hale, homeopath, concerning goldenseal

Goldenseal was known to the earliest settlers in North America, who learned of its use from the Native Americans. The first printed mention of goldenseal's native use was by the Jesuit LeMoyne, who learned of it from the Iroquois around 1650. It was also used by the Crow, Cherokee, Meskwaki, Seminole, and Blackfoot. It was an article of trade between tribes that had access to its habitat and those that did not, being used for dye as well as medicine. Many of these uses were recorded not in early medical texts, but in lay books intended as home prescribers for the pioneers

BOX 12.1
THE NAMES OF GOLDENSEAL

Hydrastis canadensis, the Latin name for goldenseal, means "a Canadian plant that accomplishes water," indicating its ability to stimulate the flow of mucus.

English: eye balm; eye root; goldenseal; ground raspberry; Indian dye; Indian paint; Indian turmeric; jaundice root; Ohio curcuma; orange root; yellow eye; yellow puccoon; yellow root

Czech: vodilka kanadska

Danish: hydrastis rod

French: hydrastis

German: Canadische gelbwurzel, goldisegelwurzel, hydrastisrhizom

Italian: idraste

Latin: *Hydrastis canadensis*

Polish: gorzknik

Russian: zeltokorien kandskii

Swedish: hydrastisrot

(Veninga and Zaricor, 1976). Box 12.2 shows some Native American uses for goldenseal.

EARLY COLONIAL MEDICINE

Goldenseal was introduced into American medical literature by Dr. Benjamin Smith Barton of Philadelphia in the first American systematic account of medicinal plants, *Collections for an Essay Towards a Materia Medica of the United States,* published in 1798. Barton made reference to the Cherokee use of the plant for cancers (probably skin cancers), and mentioned its use among the colonists as a bitter tonic and an eyewash. It is still used by naturopathic physicians as a bitter tonic and eyewash today, two centuries later. Barton called it a "pure tonic" and an "alterative in disease conditions of the mucous

---

BOX 12.2
NATIVE AMERICAN USES FOR GOLDENSEAL

acne	pelvic bleeding
catarrh	skin cancer
dye for clothing	skin ulcers
eczema	sore and inflamed eyes
indigestion	wound healing
liver problems	

(Source: Veninga and Zaricor, 1976)

membranes" (Barton, 1798). Constantine Rafinesque, whose life and work I described in Chapter 2, also wrote about goldenseal and was influential in spreading its use to the various medical sects of the nineteenth century.

Thompsonian Herbalism

A major force in introducing the general public to the use of goldenseal was the Thompsonian school of herbalism, which flourished in the first half of the nineteenth century. Samuel Thompson was a lay herbalist from New England, often at odds with the Regular school, members of which had him imprisoned for a time on false charges of killing a patient in his care. Thompson developed a simple system of medicine and created a movement that swept the country, especially the farm regions of the recently settled Midwest, from Ohio to Missouri. Millions of Americans learned simple herbal self-care from Thompson's books and purchased herbs from him. His movement eventually evolved into the Physiomedicalist school of medicine in the second half of the nineteenth century. The Physiomedicalists followed Thompson's principles, but received formal medical training, and expanded on the number of herbs that Thompson used. The *Thompsonian Recorder*, read by millions of Americans, told of goldenseal's properties in 1932. See Box 12.3 for details.

THE HOMEOPATHIC PROVINGS OF DR. EDWIN HALE

By the mid-nineteenth century, all the schools of medicine in America were using goldenseal in one way or another. It was the Homeopathic school, however, in the person of Dr.

Edwin Hale, that did the most systematic research into its medicinal effects. As I discussed briefly in Chapter 7, homeopaths sometimes perform "provings" of medicines, taking them while healthy to see what symptoms they produce. Hale and his contemporary homeopath, Dr. Constantine Hering, did provings on hundreds of North American plants, introducing them to the homeopathic professions in both North America and Europe.

Hale's records of the North American plants take up more than 1,600 pages in two volumes of his *New Remedies* series. Hering's records of the symptoms and case studies with the various herbs take up more than 5,500 pages in his ten-volume *Guiding Symptoms of our Materia Medica*, with twenty-three pages devoted to goldenseal alone. These two physicians' clinical observations of the effects of herbs are a treasure of medical information universally overlooked by contemporary herbalists because of general ignorance of the literature of the Homeopathic school. Hale supervised the first homeopathic provings of goldenseal, used it clinically for more than twenty years, and then began writing extensively about it. Despite 150 years of medical-level goldenseal use since Hale began his experiments, his observations of its effects remain the most systematic and thorough, and the most useful for us today to learn how to use this herb. Hale begins:

> *Its general primary effect on the system when taken in medicinal quantities by a healthy person will undoubtedly be that of a nutrient tonic, i.e., it stimulates the digestive processes and increases the assimilation of food. By these means, the blood is enriched, and this blood feeds the muscular system.*
>
> (Hale, 1875)

BOX 12.3

GOLDENSEAL IN THE MEDICAL SECTS:
200 YEARS OF GOLDENSEAL IN MEDICINE

Dr. Benjamin Smith Barton
(Regular school), 1798

Bitter tonic, eyewash, alterative to mucous
membranes, skin cancer treatment

Constantine Rafinesque
(Eclectic school), 1830

Bitter tonic, diuretic, stimulant, treatment for sore
eyes, skin cancers, sores, and skin ulcers

Samuel Thompson
(Thompsonian school), 1833

Treatment for relief and removal of bowel complaints, nausea and heartburn, morning sickness,
sore eyes, and stomach problems

(The Thompsonian Recorder, 1833)

Dr. John King
(Eclectic school), 1852

Bitter tonic; treatment for alcoholism, indigestion,
sore eyes, sores, skin ulcers and chronic infections of the mucous membranes of the stomach,
intestines, and bladder

Dr. William Cook
(Physiomedicalist school), 1862

Bitter tonic; tonic for digestion, mucous membrane,
veins, uterus; treatment for bladder problems,

catarrh, chronic diarrhea, coughs, diphtheria, dysentery (second stage), eye problems, liver problems, mouth ulcers, and skin ulcers

Dr. John Scudder
(Eclectic school), 1874

Bitter tonic, digestive tonic; treatment for constipation, eye problems, uterine disorders, poor circulation, and skin disorders

Dr. Edwin Hale
(Homeopathic school), 1875

Bitter tonic, digestive and mucous membrane tonic; diuretic; urinary tract antiseptic; treatment for constipation, eye inflammation, liver problems, mouth ulcers, skin problems, and sore throat (chronic)

Dr. Eli Jones
(Eclectic and Homeopathic schools), 1911

Digestive tonic; treatment for cancer (breast and stomach), constipation, liver and gall bladder disease, and skin problems

Dr. Finley Ellingwood
(Eclectic school), 1919

Tonic stimulant, bitter tonic, digestive tonic; aid to recuperation after prolonged fever; treatment for alcoholism, breast cancer, catarrh, constipation, eczema, eye inflammation, liver congestion and gall bladder problems, menstrual irregularities, mouth ulcers, uterine complaints, and vaginal discharge

(continues)

Dr. Harvey M. Felter
(Eclectic school), 1922

Bitter tonic, mucous membrane tonic; treatment
for ear infections, skin disorders, mouth ulcers,
later stages of diarrhea and dysentery, uterine disorders, catarrh, vaginal discharge, and menstrual
irregularities

Dr. David Culbreth
(Regular school), 1927

Bitter tonic, mucous membrane tonic; diuretic;
treatment for catarrh, constipation, eye problems,
liver and gall bladder congestion, sores and ulcers,
sore throat, tonsillitis, uterine disorders, and vaginal discharge

Dr. G. Madaus
(German Regular and Homeopathic schools), 1938

Treatment for menstrual irregularities, passive uterine bleeding, and uterine fibroids

Dr. A.W. Kuts-Chereaux
(Naturopathic school), 1953

Digestive tonic, mucous membrane tonic; treatment
for catarrh, dysentery, ear problems, eye inflammations, sore throat, tonsillitis, and vaginal complaints

Dr. O.J. Carroll
(Naturopathic/Thompsonian school), 1962

General tonic, bitter tonic, mucous membrane
tonic; treatment for nasal catarrh or sinusitis

Dr. John R. Christopher
(Thompsonian/American Physiomedicalist school),
1976

> Antiseptic; bitter tonic, mucous membrane tonic,
> venous circulatory tonic; diuretic; treatment for
> constipation or eye problems

Drs. Calvin and Agatha Thrash
(American Naturopathic and Regular school), 1981

> Diuretic; treatment for eczema, skin infections
> and inflammations, ulcerative colitis, and vaginal
> infections

Drs. A.W. Priest and L.R. Priest
(British Naturopathic and Physiomedicalist schools),
1982

> Antiseptic; general tonic; mucous membrane tonic,
> venous circulatory tonic; laxative; treatment for
> skin and mucous membrane ulcers

Bitter Tonic

Hale says that, through this process of improved nutrition, goldenseal also improves the nervous system. What
Hale describes here is the action of the classic *bitter tonic,* a
famous term in the history of natural medicine. Plants or
other substances with a bitter flavor (including black coffee)
stimulate digestive secretions. When an individual is weakened because of a chronically weak digestive system, such
tonics, taken before meals for a period of time, can restore

the digestion and the strength of the system as a whole. They are taken for sluggish digestion, poor assimilation, muscular weakness, and accompanying nervous debility.

Contemporary herbalist Michael Moore describes the indications and contraindications for goldenseal thus:

- Indications: Upper intestinal tract deficiency, with dry mouth, gum problems, coated tongue, and sluggish gastric secretions.
- Contraindications: Gastric inflammation, with a moist mouth and pointed, red-tipped tongue (Moore, 1993).

Goldenseal is not unique as a bitter tonic; other plants in this book are also excellent bitter tonics, including the goldenseal substitutes mentioned in the next chapter, and boneset, discussed in Chapter 17. It is a common practice in Europe to take "bitters" before meals to improve digestion.

Mucous Membrane Tonic

Hale then captures the second key action of goldenseal: "Its primary effect on the glandular system is to excite to unusual secretion." Hale here refers to the glands of the mucous membranes, especially those in the stomach and intestines, and also the liver, which secretes bile. Normally we think of mucus as "the enemy" during an illness, but this is a misconception. During the initial stages of infection and inflammation, mucus flows freely. If the infection persists, however, the membranes become sluggish and ulcerated, and the mucus becomes thick and ropey.

We saw in Chapter 4, however, that mucus has a protective effect on the body, both mechanically as a barrier, and

immunologically because it is infused with antibodies. When
its flow becomes stagnant, these protective functions are im-
paired and secondary infections can set in. This is the patho-
logical course of affairs when, for instance, a chronic cold or
bronchitis progresses to pneumonia. Sluggish or deficient
mucous secretions in the stomach or small intestine can lead
to ulcers. Ulcerative colitis may have a similar pathology.

So when the mucous membranes have become stagnant, boggy, ulcerated, or infected, goldenseal is an ideal
remedy. It stimulates the flow of fresh, clean, and antibody-
infused mucus to fight any persistent infection and help heal
the inflamed membranes. This includes the membranes of
the bladder, ears, eyes, intestines, sinuses, stomach, urethra,
uterus, and vagina. Examine Box 12.3 and see how many
conditions of the mucous membranes have been benefited by
medical prescriptions of goldenseal in the last two centuries.
The mucus-stimulating effect of goldenseal makes it highly
versatile.

Hale wrote in the days before the discovery of germs
and the dominance of the germ-theory of disease. Thus he did
not know that constituents of goldenseal will kill bacteria on
contact. This action is doubtlessly important in the direct application of goldenseal to infected external sores or to mucous
membranes. For most of the effects listed in Box 12.3, however, the combination of bitter tonic and mucous membrane
stimulant effects is at work, rather than antibiotic effects.

Contemporary traditional Appalachian herbalist A.L.
Tommie Bass has referred to goldenseal as the "King and
Queen" of the herbs that the Good Lord put in the ground.
We might call goldenseal's bitter tonic properties the "King,"
and its mucous membrane tonic properties the "Queen." We
have plenty of other bitter tonic herbs—"Kings"—and a

handful of mucous membrane tonics—"Queens"—but gold-enseal is the only plant we have that marries them together. This is its uniqueness and power, and the reason for its universal popularity on this continent since before the founding of the United States.

Dose and Applications

Hale, like the Eclectics after him, did not recommend large doses of goldenseal, with the maximum dose being about half a dropperful of the tincture or tea. Doses of three to five drops, in water, were quite effective for most of the uses listed in Box 12.3. Modern consumers waste of lot of expensive goldenseal by taking larger doses—usually inappropriately—for colds and flu. Eye infections, one of the classic applications of goldenseal, require more diluted applications for a wash—fifteen to twenty drops of tea in a pint of water. Hale also introduced the use of goldenseal tea (not tincture) as a spray in an atomizer. This is, of course, an effective application for a sore throat, but he also used it in cases of bronchitis, saying that a small amount of it will inadvertently be inhaled and will benefit the infected bronchi. Some specific conditions for which Hale used goldenseal include:

- acid indigestion (low doses)
- dysentery (later stages)
- eye inflammation (diluted tea)
- hemorrhoids (use enemas at night)
- liver congestion and jaundice (tea)
- mouth ulcers (tea)
- sluggish digestion (tea)
- sore throat (gargle plus internal use for
  chronic stage)

BOX 12.4

DR. EDWIN HALE'S METHODS OF APPLICATION OF GOLDENSEAL

atomizer	powder
douche	syringe
enema	tea
lotion	tincture

wash (one part tincture to ten parts water)

- stomach ulcer
- ulcerative colitis (not during acute phase)
- urinary tract infection (acute or chronic)
- uterine and vaginal mucus discharges (douche plus internal use)

GYNECOLOGICAL USE

Many of the practitioners listed in Box 12.3 have used gold-enseal to treat gynecological problems; this very effective use has been all but forgotten today. When the mucous membranes of the female reproductive tract are chronically congested, with a discharge, goldenseal may be applied as a douche and also taken orally. Some practitioners, from Hale on, have used goldenseal to treat painful menstruation. German homeopaths learned its use from Hale, and it became widely accepted in Germany as a remedy for painful menstruation or for bleeding from uterine fibroids (Madaus, 1938).

Several German formulas are:

For painful menstruation (when the general indications for goldenseal are present):

goldenseal *(Hydrastis canadensis)*
black haw *(Viburnum prunifolium)*

Twenty to forty drops of standard tincture (1:5) in warm water, repeated daily for eight days before the expected period.

For passive bleeding and fibroids:

goldenseal *(Hydrastis canadensis)*
witch hazel *(Hamamelis virginiana)*
cinnamon

Fifteen to twenty drops of standard tincture (1:5) in warm water every three hours.

SUMMARY OF TRADITIONAL USE AND CAUTIONS

As is evident in Box 12.3, goldenseal can be used to treat a wide range of medical conditions. The overall indication for its use as a tonic is poor digestion, general weakness, obstinate constipation, and the chronically congested state of the mucous membranes. Most of the physicians listed cautioned against its use in acute inflammation, recommending it instead for "subacute" and chronic states, distinctions that I will explain in detail in Table 13.2. It may also be used externally on infected wounds, sores, and ulcers. Note that none of these physicians used it to treat colds and flu, which are probably its most common uses today. Physicians have traditionally cautioned against its use when the mucous membranes or skin eruptions are dry; moist and congested membranes are the key indication. Hale also cautioned against large doses or prolonged use, which can injure and disrupt the normal functioning of the digestive tract—the very condition that it can cure in low doses.

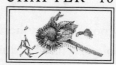

CHAPTER 13

SCIENTIFIC RESEARCH: BERBERINE AND HYDRASTINE

A search of contemporary scientific research turns up not a single clinical trial of goldenseal for any condition. While this may seem odd for such a popular medicine, there are two reasons for the poverty of scientific investigation: (1) the conventional school of medicine never really used goldenseal to any great extent and thus is unfamiliar with it, and (2) methods for synthesizing its constituents have been known for so long that a patent cannot be obtained for them. Potential patentability of a new drug is usually the driving economic force behind scientific research into plants.

Most of the modern research into "goldenseal" has been into its constituent *berberine*. Table 13.1 shows some of the chemical constituents of goldenseal. Some scientists and contemporary herbal writers state outright that the activity of goldenseal is due to its berberine content. The statement is quite unscientific, because the basic research to determine the separate clinical effects of its constituents has never been performed. We have dozens of plants containing berberine, a few of which I'll describe later in Chapter 15, but none of them—even those containing more berberine than goldenseal—have attained the reputation as the "King and Queen" of herbs. That reputation is due to goldenseal's unique combination of constituents, not to berberine alone.

One Eclectic writer held that *hydrastine* is solely responsible for some effects of goldenseal (Felter, 1922), and others even describe the use of extracted hydrastine in the place of goldenseal (Ellingwood, 1919; Felter, 1922). Later pharmaceutical writers also held that goldenseal's main action was due to hydrastine rather than berberine (Osol and Farrar, 1947). Other constituents are also important. The Eclectic pharmacist John Uri Lloyd reported research in 1898 showing that a goldenseal extract with both the berberine and the hydrastine removed still had medicinal effects. The other components have an astringent, drying effect, which can cause unpleasant side effects if goldenseal is taken in high doses. Virtually all the research described in this chapter was done with berberine rather than goldenseal itself.

Table 13.1   The Alkaloid Constituents of Goldenseal

Berberine	2 to 4 percent
Hydrastine	2 to 3 percent
Canadine	< 1 percent

(Source: *Merck Index*, Eleventh Edition, 1989)

ANTIBIOTIC EFFECTS OF BERBERINE

Goldenseal today has a wide reputation as an "herbal antibiotic," based on scientific research and the clinical use of isolated berberine, most often in the form of berberine sulfate. Box 13.1 shows a list of organisms which berberine sulfate can kill or neutralize in a petri dish. When goldenseal is used topically—put directly onto an infected wound or ulcer—the berberine in it may have such an effect on the microorganisms in the wound. From research such as this, it is enticing to conclude that goldenseal and other berberine-containing plants taken internally act in the body the same way that pharmaceutical antibiotics do, to kill or inhibit bacteria. However, clinical research actually indicates otherwise.

First of all, in humans berberine is very poorly absorbed in the small intestine (Bhide et al, 1969). Four hundred milligrams of berberine sulfate, the amount contained in about twenty-six capsules of goldenseal powder—more than you would want to take in a day, I assure you—causes blood levels of berberine to rise to only about one-two-hundredth of the level required to kill the bacteria shown in Box 13.1 (Bensky and Gamble, 1986). Thus, berberine itself does not act as a systemic antibiotic; goldenseal, which contains only a small percentage of berberine, cannot do so either—at least not due to its berberine content.

Berberine is excreted through the urine in humans (Chopra et al, 1932), so it could conceivably have some antibiotic effect on kidney or urinary tract infections via the concentrated urine. Goldenseal was used for these conditions by American physicians of the last century, but we have no scientific evidence to support that action.

That leaves open the question as to whether berberine or goldenseal act as antibiotics against pathogenic bacteria

BOX 13.1

ORGANISMS KILLED OR CONTROLLED BY BERBERINE SULFATE *IN VITRO*

BACTERIA

Bacillus cerus
B. subtilis
Corynebacterium
  diphtheria
Enterobacter aerogenes
Erwinia carotavora
Escherichia coli
Klebsiella spp.
K. Pneumoniae
Mycobacterium
  tuberculosis

Proteus spp.
Pseudomonas
  mangiferae
Salmonella paratyphi
S. typhimurium
Shighella boydii
Staphylococcus
  aureus
Streptococcus pyrogenes
Vibrio cholerae
Xanthomonas citri

FUNGI

Candida albicans
C. utilis
Cryptococcus neoformans
Microsporum gypseum

Saccharomyces cerevisiae
Sporothrix schenkii
Trichophyton
  mentagrophytes

PARASITES

Entamoeba histolytica
Giardia lamblia

Leishmania donovani
Trichomonas vaginalis

(Sources: Amin et al, 1969; Choudry et al, 1972; Ghosh, 1983; Gupta, 1975; Johnson et al, 1952; Subbaiah and Amin, 1967)

within the intestine. Berberine sulfate is used clinically in Asia to treat diarrheal infections, and antibiotic effects might seem a natural explanation. In one double-blind placebo-controlled trial, 400-mg doses of berberine sulfate were given orally to men with *E. coli*-induced diarrhea. The group receiving the berberine had a forty-eight-percent reduction in stool volumes; forty-two percent of the men in the group stopped having watery stools within twenty-four hours, compared with twenty percent in the control group, which received only a placebo. The results are typical of treatment of diarrhea with berberine. This trial is frequently cited by herbal companies as "proof" that berberine-containing plants kill bacteria in the intestine, even though the authors of that trial reached the opposite conclusion. They found that bacterial counts in the patients were unchanged (Rabbani et al., 1987).

The berberine could have been acting through mechanisms other than killing the bacteria to control the infections:

- It could have acted to strengthen the integrity of the mucous membrane, or to increase the flow of antibody-laden mucus to the site of infection, an action consistent with its traditional use.
- It could have acted to prevent attachment of the organisms to the intestinal walls without killing them. Several trials have shown that berberine prevents other kinds of bacteria from adhering to cells, including streptococcus (Sun et al., 1988a, b).
- It could have neutralized the bacterial toxins while leaving the bacteria intact; several experiments have shown that berberine can reduce symptoms in toxin-induced diarrhea, even when the bacteria that normally secrete the toxins are not present

(Sabir et al, 1977; Swabb et al, 1981; Zhu and Ahrens, 1982).

- Other researchers have suggested that it may inhibit the metabolism of certain organisms, resulting in decreased formation of toxins (Akhter et al, 1977; Amin et al, 1969; Sabir et al, 1977).

None of these scientific hypotheses have been supported by specific studies. Research into another condition may shed light on the action of berberine in diarrheal infections. We saw that goldenseal has been used ever since the time of the early Native Americans as an eyewash for eye infections. Berberine extracts are used the same way in Asia, and recent research into viral eye infections there showed it to have profound effects against infection by the trachoma virus (Babbar et al, 1982; Mohan et al, 1982; Sabir et al, 1976).

Chlamydia trachomatis, commonly known as trachoma, infects the eyes of as many as a half-billion people worldwide, especially in the tropics, and results in blindness in as many as two million people every year. Even with antibiotic therapy, the infection can last as long as a year. In the typical course, the membranes around the eye become ulcerated and scarred, interfering with the function of the tear ducts. Several clinical trials have demonstrated that berberine sulfate is superior to the conventional pharmaceutical drugs used to treat this condition (Babbar et al, 1982; Sabir et al, 1976). In the Babbar trial, patients infected with trachoma were divided into three groups. One received berberine eye drops; the second received berberine and sulfacetamide drops, the antibiotic most often used to treat this condition. The third group received the antibiotic only. After three weeks, the results showed that the antibiotic-only group appeared to have the best clinical results, although all three groups showed improvement. However, the virus was still present in the eye tissues of all the subjects in this group, and relapse of the disease was likely in all. Groups one and two, who had taken berberine sulfate, had more modest initial symptomatic results, but the virus was eliminated from the eyes in 100 percent of the subjects.

Seeking to identify the mechanism by which berberine killed the virus in the trial, the researchers experimented with berberine and viral cultures. It had no direct antiviral effect. The authors suggest that berberine acts by "stimulating some protective mechanism in the host."

PROTECTIVE FACTORS:
THE HEALING POWER OF SNOT

Just what are these "protective factors" in the body that might have been stimulated by berberine to kill 100 percent of the virus in 100 percent of the patients in the trial above? Our culture has become enamored of the germ theory of disease, and of the power of antibiotics, but actual illness does not fit the popular model. An infection requires two things: (1) an infectious agent and (2) fertile ground in the body. Most people who are exposed to a germ do not get sick, because they do not supply fertile ground for the infection to take hold. This is why a flu epidemic can sweep through a town, and usually not more than a third of the population is infected, though virtually everyone is exposed.

One of the most potent weapons in the immune system is found infused in the mucous secretions of the respiratory, digestive, and urinary tracts, and in the saliva and tears. This weapon is the *immunoglobulin A* antibody, called *IgA*. We saw in Chapter 4 that antibodies act to neutralize or destroy potential invaders. This particular form of antibody is super-charged; it contains twice the number of binding sites that most other antibodies have. IgA is specialized to protect the body at the surface. It can prevent potential invaders and even bacterial toxins from attaching to the cells of the sur-face membranes, and, if they do attach there, evoke a killing immune system response against them.

The mucus, tears, and saliva (and mother's milk) are saturated with these IgA antibodies. There may be millions of different IgA-type antibodies in the mucus—the same kind that are contained in the plasma and tissues. The highest amounts at any time will be antibodies to infections that are currently active. Thus, mucus is not "the enemy" in an infec-tion, but is a sophisticated, genetically engineered antibiotic paste that is tailored to whatever infection is current. People make a mistake by taking decongestants during a cold or flu; they are actually prolonging their illness. Taking high amounts of goldenseal in the early stages of a cold can have the same effect, drying the membranes. A better strategy, endorsed by all schools of medicine, is to drink plenty of liquids to thin the mucus and ensure that it flows freely.

We saw that, in traditional medical use, goldenseal was indicated for subacute and chronic infections of the mucous membranes, but not for the acute stage—"not until the fever has subsided," according to Hale. Table 13.2 shows the condi-tion of the mucous membranes during each of these stages. The pathology could be the same for dozens of individually named conditions: nasal catarrh, sinusitis, chronic bronchitis, duodenal ulcer, dysentery, ulcerative colitis, urinary tract ca-tarrh, chronic vaginal infection, eye infection, etc.

Table 13.2 The Pathology of the Stages of Infection of the Mucous Membranes

Acute:	Mucus flows freely, mechanically washing away invaders and/or "tagging" them with IgA antibodies; inflammation and swelling of the tissues walls off invaders to prevent penetration and floods the area with immune system cells; any agent penetrating to the level of the lymphatics triggers humoral and cell-mediated immunity.
Subacute:	The initial fever or inflammation subsides; the area may become congested with the boggy by-products of the immune system battle. The process that initially walled off the area in a protective way now blocks out the influx of immune system components. Ulceration, scarring, and other lesions begin to develop. Secondary infections may start to set in. Meanwhile, the body is accumulating high levels of antibodies to any new infectious agent, but they cannot get to the congested tissues.
Chronic:	Ulceration and scarring of the membranes occurs; membranes become dry and cracked as mucous secretions are blocked or deranged. Bleeding may occur. Secondary infections may occur due to weakened circulation of immune system components.

Taking goldenseal or berberine internally will not directly kill or inhibit bacteria or other infectious agents in most of these conditions. What they will do, as we saw in the section on traditional medicine, is excite the mucous membranes "to unusual secretion." In doing so, in the second and third stages of the pathology, the fresh and abundant mucous can soothe, clean, disinfect, and heal the tissues. Taking goldenseal too early in the process—especially in high doses—can have negative effects. It may:

- exhaust the mucous glands by overstimulating them, and dry the membranes (two to three goldenseal capsules has a distinct drying effect on the membrane)
- inhibit the healthy inflammatory reaction, weakening the immune system response, and prolonging the illness
- weaken the digestive system (see the section that describes adverse reactions to high doses of goldenseal)

So berberine may have worked in the trachoma cases by healing and restoring the normal function of the membranes around the eye, allowing the free flow of IgA-laden tears to do its virus-killing work. The same process could account for its action in the intestine. Infections that cause watery diarrhea occur in tiny, almost microscopic pits that line the small intestine. These "crypts of Leiberkühn" are like small wells with narrow tops. Within them are cells that secrete watery fluid to help dissolve and absorb nutrients from the intestine. The fluid is almost immediately reabsorbed. About two quarts of such fluid is secreted each day in the normal intestine, but during infection of the secreting cells up to fifteen quarts can be lost in conditions such as cholera. Death can occur from dehydration. Such an infection requires that the bacteria or its toxins penetrate the crypts. Also within the crypts, however, are mucous glands. Berberine, again by stimulating these glands "to unusual secretion," can flood the crypt with mucous-carried antibodies to the bacteria and/or its toxin, killing them or preventing them from adhering to the wall of the crypt.

Berberine also has an "antisecretory" effect on the uninfected intestine, tending to reduce these watery secretions of the small intestine. In a trial with pigs, this effect was seen in the small intestine of normal, uninfected animals (Zhu and Ahrens, 1983). Such secretions are important to digestion. They keep the intestines moist, wash potential pathogens out of the nooks and crannies of the intestine, and purify the extracellular fluid.

GOLDENSEAL DOES NOT DISRUPT NORMAL BOWEL FLORA

One side effect of the myth that goldenseal is an antibiotic is the belief that it might, like conventional antibiotics, disrupt the balance of normal bacteria in the intestine. This action is responsible for some of the minor or serious side effects of antibiotics. We have no evidence, either from traditional use or from scientific experiments, that either berberine or goldenseal can cause this problem. In fact, in the Rabbani trial described previously in this chapter, the berberine did not even kill the pathogenic bacteria in the intestine. I first heard about this possibility in the mid-1980s. I've been looking for a single case report of this effect ever since and have never heard of one.

OTHER EFFECTS OF GOLDENSEAL

Stimulant Effects

The Eclectic and Physiomedicalist schools of herbalism also classified goldenseal as a stimulant (Cook, 1869; Ellingwood, 1919). This may be due to its constituent, hydrastine, which has effects on the central nervous system, antagonizing GABA receptors in the nerve synapses (Qian and Dowling,

1994). The net effect is stimulation of the nerves. Ellingwood compared the action of hydrastis to that of strychnine, which, in medicinal doses, causes contraction and increases the tone of the muscles (Ellingwood, 1919). Felter noted that the clinical effect of reducing vaginal bleeding may be due to this effect of hydrastine constricting the muscles in the uterus. Berberine also acts as a central-nervous-system stimulant in normal medicinal doses, and as a depressant in large, experimental doses in animals (Bensky and Gamble, 1986). Depressant effects have not been noted in humans (Yamahara, 1976).

An uncomfortable overstimulation of the nervous system is possible with medicinal doses of goldenseal. One of the first clients I saw when I began practicing herbalism in Taos, New Mexico, in 1978 was a woman, in the fourth day of a cold, who had tension and tremors throughout her body. She appeared very excited, and not only were her hands shaking, but her entire torso appeared to be trembling slightly. She had been taking large doses of goldenseal—two to three capsules four times a day for four days. Remember that, traditionally, physicians have used about half a dropperful three or four times a day. She had a slight build and did not weigh more than 110 pounds, so the amount she took was far more goldenseal than she would have needed—probably ten times as much—even if it had been the right herb for her condition and constitution, which it was not. We stopped the goldenseal, and the tremors promptly went away by the next day.

Abortive Effects

The stimulant effect that causes constriction of the uterine muscles may also cause abortion, or at least uterine contractions. Decoctions of certain berberine-containing plants have been employed in folk medicine as abortifacients, oxytocics, or antifertility agents (Farnsworth et al, 1975). Requests for herbal abortions are common for many contemporary herbalists in North America; I know of herbalists who supervise abortions as often as once a week. Goldenseal is sometimes used as part of the herbal protocol, after preparation with other herbs for several weeks.

In the only such case I have observed, the herbal protocol failed; the goldenseal (ten capsules) caused abdominal rather than uterine cramping, and the woman vomited up the capsules after a short while. I don't wish to imply that goldenseal can be taken safely in pregnancy—sensitive pregnancies might be much more vulnerable—but to demonstrate that miscarriage is probably not a large public health problem. I am assured by several professional herbalists that goldenseal does sometimes initiate uterine contractions. As a further note, herbal abortion can be quite uncomfortable; you are basically poisoning your entire body with herbal drugs in order to affect the uterus. My "herbal mothers"— the women who first taught me herbalism—cautioned that a clinical abortion was quicker, less traumatic, and safer, and in nearly twenty years of practice, I have never seen anything to change my mind on the subject.

OTHER BERBERINE RESEARCH

We saw above that berberine's antibiotic effects have been extensively researched. Berberine has attracted other research attention, especially in Asia, where it is used as a "poor man's" antibiotic. It has been used for centuries, either isolated or in berberine-containing plants, in both Ayurvedic (East Indian) and traditional Chinese medicine.

Anti-Inflammatory Effects

Berberine has an anti-inflammatory effect, possibly through the same intracellular mechanism as aspirin (Xuan et al., 1994; Sabir et al., 1978; Akhter et al., 1977). This may contribute to goldenseal's ability to reduce inflammation of mucous membranes. In traditional medical systems, berberine-containing plants are considered "cooling." A study in animals found that berberine lowered fever three times as efficiently as aspirin. It is not clear what dose of a berberine-containing plant a human would require to get the same effect, but berberine-containing plants are not known to dramatically reduce fevers. If fact, Hale considered that goldenseal was contraindicated during fever, and should be given only when fever and acute inflammation have subsided to the subacute or chronic stage.

Anti-Ulcer Effects

Berberine has also demonstrated mild anti-ulcer effects in mice, supporting the traditional use of berberine-containing herbs in the treatment of ulcers (Yamahara, 1976). The investigators in this trial used berberine isolated from the Chinese coptis plant, which I will describe in Chapter 15 as a goldenseal substitute.

Diarrhea Case Details

The use of berberine best supported by science is as a remedy for intestinal infections. A number of clinical reports from India in the late 1960s, cited in the section on antibiotics above, showed that berberine is useful in treating E. coli, cholera, and giardia. The Rabbani trial in 1987 was the first well-controlled trial of berberine in a specific intestinal infection (Rabbani et al, 1987). This trial, using 400-mg doses of berberine sulfate, showed better effects against *E. coli* than against *V. cholerae*. In a trial in China, a dose of 100 mg of berberine sulfate taken four times daily was no more effective than a placebo (Khin-Maung et al, 1985), so the dosage may be critical. The lowest dose shown to be effective for diarrhea was 150 mg of berberine sulfate per day — the equivalent of about five grams of goldenseal powder, or ten capsules per day (Kamsat, 1967). The 400-mg dose is equivalent to about twenty-six goldenseal capsules, and this dose is sometimes taken three times a day! This is obviously not a feasible treatment, and would begin to produce the adverse effects I will describe in the next chapter. Note, however, that these are very serious, and potentially life-threatening intestinal infections. Less serious infections were routinely treated with smaller doses of goldenseal by the physicians of the last century.

I personally supervised treatment of a case of pathogenic *E. coli* infection in Colorado caused by contaminated apple juice. At the first onset of bloody diarrhea, at the end of a three-day fever, the adult patient began taking twenty drops of a tincture of three berberine-containing plants (Oregon grape, barberry, and goldenseal) in warm water every two or three hours. All bleeding stopped within twenty-four hours. Note that *E. coli* infection can be a medical emergency in children, who should be hospitalized or supervised by a physician.

Parasites

Berberine may also be effective in treating parasitic infections. Some writers unfortunately have stated that it may be an effective treatment for the amoebic parasite *Entamoeba histolytica*. This is based on a 1967 study of hamsters, in which infection with *E. histolytica* was successfully avoided by *pretreatment* with berberine. Doses of berberine were also given along with the amoebic infection, and shortly afterward. The dose was 5 mg per kg of animal weight—about the equivalent of the 400-mg adult dose of berberine sulfate used successfully in the diarrhea trials. There is no such evidence that berberine has this clinical effect in humans, and even if it did, you would have to take it *before* the infection to get the same results. Three such doses in a human, which would match the dose in the hamsters, would require eighty goldenseal capsules over an eight-hour period. As I mentioned above, I've seen ten-capsule doses cause abdominal cramping and vomiting. *E. histolytica* is a potentially serious infection that can spread beyond the digestive tract to damage organs in the body; it requires medical supervision, even if you are trying a natural remedy. I have seen cases in which it was effectively eradicated using the herb Chinese wormwood *(Artemisia annua)* over a period of months, along with other treatments, as confirmed by stool analysis by the supervising physician.

Other trials have shown that berberine sulfate can eradicate the giardia parasite (Choudry et al, 1972; Gupta, 1975). The 400 mg dose of berberine adjusted downward for the weight of the individual child, was given to patients aged one to fourteen years old who were infected with giardia. The treatment was compared to the conventional treatment with the drug metronidazole (Flagyl). Berberine was about as effective as the drug, but with almost no side effects. Flagyl has potentially serious side effects, such as nerve damage and cancer, and is often devastating to the natural balance of the digestive tract. It is questionable whether these results can be repeated with whole herbs rather than isolated berberine because of the volumes of herbs required and the side effects that appear at such high doses.

Immune System Stimulation

Some popular writers describe goldenseal as an immune system stimulant, citing several scientific studies as proof. How relevant these trials are to humans taking berberine-containing plants is questionable, however. One trial in animals demonstrated that berberine increases blood flow through the spleen (Sabir, 1971). The spleen is a large lymphatic organ, right next to the stomach, that filters blood rather than lymph. The amount of blood flowing through it is variable, depending on physiological conditions, especially the need for blood in the muscles. Spleen function can vary widely between humans and animals. Many animals have a muscular capsule around the spleen to control its volume, but humans do not, so the berberine results in animals do not necessarily apply to humans. As we saw above, the way a drug is processed in the body is often quite different between animals and humans. For instance, berberine is not excreted in the urine of test animals, while significant amounts of it reach the urine and the urinary tract in humans (Department of National Health and Welfare, 1989). And finally, spleen blood flow is not a significant indicator of immunity.

One other animal trial showed that berberine activated macrophages of animals in test-tube experiments (Kumazawa, 1984). Such abstract research demonstrates nothing about the activity of goldenseal itself, much less that of berberine-containing plants.

Anti-Cancer Effects

Goldenseal has been used traditionally in the treatment of cancers, especially skin cancers (Barton, 1798; Hale, 1875) and breast cancer (Jones, 1911). Modern screening trials have shown that berberine may have some antitumor activity (Duke, 1985), but remember that these trials using concentrated extracts in petri dishes and animal screens often have no relevance to the human oral use of herbs. Even by the 1920s, however, the Eclectics advised against relying on goldenseal for the treatment of cancer (Felter, 1922), and modern treatments for the two cancers mentioned are more effective than the traditional ones. Surgical removal of skin cancers, for instance, is more precise and less likely to disfigure the skin than herbal treatments. Goldenseal may be beneficial to the overall health of a cancer patient who otherwise exhibits the indications for its use, but it is not a direct treatment for any known cancer, and is not used that way today by herbalists who treat cancer.

SUMMARY

Goldenseal as a whole herb has not been tested in clinical trials. Its alkaloid constituent, berberine, has been more widely studied. The antibiotic effects of berberine may have some effect in topical, intestinal, and urinary tract infections, but do not have systemic antibiotic effects. Berberine and plants containing it may act against infection by stimulating the natural protective factors in the mucous membranes rather than killing organisms directly. Goldenseal itself contains only a small amount of berberine, and its other constituents, which many herbalists consider to be more important than berberine, have not been studied clinically.

CHAPTER 14

How to Use (and Not Use) Goldenseal

Goldenseal is an endangered plant with a greatly inflated price. Most people who purchase it do so for colds and flu, or to "beat" a drug test. In the first case, it may actually make the condition worse, and in the second, it is useless. Thus it is more important to describe how *not* to use goldenseal than how to use it.

Colds and Flu

In my experience, both selling herbs at retail and seeing patients in the clinic, not even ten percent of the goldenseal use in the U.S. is clinically appropriate. When someone pops large amounts of goldenseal "for a cold," especially in its early stages, they are wasting both their money and an endangered plant. People in our culture are conditioned to think "I need an antibiotic" when they have a cold. I explained in the last two chapters that goldenseal's reputation as an antibiotic — for anything other than topical applications and possibly intestinal infections — is not supported by either traditional use or by modern science. Taking goldenseal in the early stages of a cold or flu can actually make the condition worse. The reason: It is drying to the mucous membranes.

Mucus is Not the Enemy

We saw in Chapters 4 and 13 that mucous membranes are part of the first layer of the immune system's defensive barriers, and that the mucus itself is saturated with antibodies to bacteria, viruses, and other invaders. Goldenseal, especially in capsules or tincture doses of more than about fifteen drops, can dry the mucous membranes in an acute situation, and thereby inhibit the immune system. Your condition may seem to get better because of the drying effect, but it actually inhibits the natural defenses against whatever bug has got you. Goldenseal may be appropriate on the third or fourth day of a cold or flu, if there is any fear of a bacterial infection setting in. At that stage, in smaller doses, goldenseal will restore a healthy flow of mucus to the stagnant membranes.

Large Doses of Goldenseal

Goldenseal provides its internal benefits in small doses — ten to fifteen drops of a tincture or fluid extract in a glass of water — and does its work in a few days to a week. Larger doses or longer duration can begin to cause side effects. Here is how Dr. Edwin Hale described the effects of taking too much goldenseal:

*The increased digestive power gives way to indiges-
tion; the increased power of assimilation to deficient
nutrition; and apparent strength to real debility. . . .
the natural secretion [of the mucous membranes] is
at first increased; then it becomes abnormal in quantity and quality. At first clear, white, and transpar-
ent, it becomes yellow, or thick, green, and even
bloody, and nearly always tenacious. . . . The dis-
tance traversed by the primary mucous flux passes
from simple increase of mucus, to erosion and ulceration. Its secondary effects are exhaustion and destruction of the glandular sources of the mucus—a
condition in which the mucous surface is dry, glazed,
and its functions destroyed.*

(Hale, 1875)

The digestive tract is especially susceptible to such
effects, and individuals who take goldenseal for their colds
are usually injuring their stomach and intestines instead of
helping their cold.

OTHER EFFECTS OF LARGE DOSES   I described two cases
in Chapter 13 in which goldenseal induced central nervous
system tremors or nausea in patients who had taken large
doses—from forty capsules over four days to ten capsules in
a single dose. An associate of mine took large doses of a vac-
uum-concentrated goldenseal extract for a cold, and was up
all night vomiting. This wasn't just coincidence, because he
tried it another time and got the same results.

SUPPRESSION OF DIARRHEA

Goldenseal, in small doses, is an excellent treatment for the later stages of diarrhea or dysentery. In the early stages, as in the early stages of a cold, it is important not to suppress the secretions of the intestinal mucosa when they are doing their job. They not only combat infectious agents with their IgA antibodies, but they wash toxins out of the intestine.

FALSE RUMORS ABOUT GOLDENSEAL

Toxicity

Several contemporary herbal books say that goldenseal, in large doses, can cause convulsions. This appears to be based on comments in the Eclectic literature (Ellingwood, 1919; Felter, 1922) regarding animal experiments that used large experimental doses of goldenseal. Both of these texts later say that such an effect has never been observed in humans. Before you could assimilate such a dose, you would vomit.

Drug Testing

A rumor has circulated among drug users in the U.S. that goldenseal will mask the presence of drug residues in the urine. No evidence of such an effect exists, either from traditional use or from modern science. One journal article states that goldenseal with neither mask the presence of opiates nor flush them from the system (Ostrenga and Perry, 1975). The magazine *High Times*, a pro-drug publication, has stated repeatedly that *no* known substances help to thwart drug-analysis machines (Montague, 1986). Author and botanical scholar Steve Foster suggests that the rumor has its basis in an early-twentieth-century novel by pharmacist John Uri Lloyd (Foster, 1989).

I've heard a new rumor this year that drug testing laboratories are now routinely screening urine samples for the presence of hydrastine, an alkaloid component of goldenseal. If they find it, they assume that the subject is trying to hide something, and run the most sensitive, expensive test they have. I hope that the rumor stops this useless waste of goldenseal.

FORMS OF GOLDENSEAL

Goldenseal is most often available in tinctures, fluid extracts, and powdered capsules. See Chapter 11 for an explanation of each of these forms. The dose for the tincture is ten to fifteen drops, repeated three or four times a day. For the fluid extract, use a smaller dose. As I explained above, this is not a "more is better" type of herb. You won't need more than a single capsule of the powder as a dose. Break it open and stir it into some warm water.

You can also make a tea from the powder. A highly diluted tea may be used as an eyewash, or a stronger tea for application to cold sores, skin ulcers, or infected eczema. The tea does not contain the constituent hydrastine, which is only alcohol-soluble.

CHAPTER 15

GOLDENSEAL SUBSTITUTES

Berberis [barberry] acts much like hydrastis [gold-enseal] and could be employed for many of the uses of that scarce and high-priced drug so far as the berberine effects are concerned.

Dr. Harvey Felter

I have already stated that goldenseal populations have become endangered and are extinct in some regions where the plant used to grow freely. I also described in Chapter 14 how it is often used inappropriately as an "antibiotic" for colds and flu. Demand for goldenseal has made it one of our most expensive plants. By learning about the herbs in this chapter, you will discover less expensive plants that may be more appropriate for your condition, and you'll be able to save the goldenseal for the conditions that it excels in curing.

BERBERINE-CONTAINING HERBS

Most of the research that is popularly associated with goldenseal has actually been into its constituent, berberine. A number of other plants contain berberine in medicinal quantities (one of them, coptis, actually contains more berberine than does goldenseal). Table 15.1 lists the situations in which these plants can best be used in place of goldenseal. All these plants, like goldenseal, have a characteristic bitter flavor and may be used as *bitter tonics*—a term I explained in Chapter 14. They may be taken as teas, tinctures, or powdered herb in warm water. Don't take berberine-containing plants during pregnancy. This caution applies to most plants containing alkaloids, including tobacco and coffee.

Potential Toxicity

Rumors are circulating in scientific and regulatory circles that berberine may be toxic. In 1996, the committee of the European Union that regulates drugs placed barberry *(Berberis vulgaris)* in a table of "Herbal Drugs with Serious Risks Without Any Accepted Benefit" because it contains berberine. This recommendation is so out of line with the long traditional use of barberry and other berberine-containing herbs that it must be taken with a grain of salt. The "serious risks" may refer to animal trials or human incidents using large amounts of isolated berberine. The lack of "accepted benefit" may reflect the fact that these plants have not been studied in formal clinical trials, as is common with most medicinal plants.

In a computer search of the MEDLINE and TOX-LINE databases of the U.S. National Library of Medicine, I was able to find only a single report of potential adverse effects of the berberis species, berberine-containing plants, or berberine itself. This was a study performed in China that showed that berberine can adversely affect the treatment of

TABLE 15.1   GOLDENSEAL SUBSTITUTES

Colds and flu	Oregon grape root, and many of the herbs named in Chapters 16–19. Goldenseal is not effective in these conditions.
Later stage of cold, with bacterial infection of the mucous membranes	no good substitute
Topical infections	berberine-containing herbs such as barberry, Oregon grape root, or coptis
Bitter tonic	berberine-containing herbs, or such herbs as yellow dock or dandelion
Eye infections	berberine-containing herbs
Gum infections	no good substitute
Intestinal infections	berberine-containing herbs
Mucous membrane tonic	yerba mansa, either alone or in combination with berberine-containing herbs

newborn infants with prenatal liver disease (Chan, 1993). I assume that this is not a risk for the general public or for contemporary herbalists or general-practice physicians, because such an infant would be hospitalized in this country. It does support traditional cautions about using berberine-containing plants in pregnancy, however.

In a recent review of herbs toxic to the liver, two French physicians state only that barberry has been "suggested" as potentially hepatotoxic (toxic to the liver), with no specific clinical evidence. He cites Vulto and De Smet (1988) as a source, but states that no case has been confirmed, and that the problem, if there is one, is rare (Larrey and Pageaux, 1995). Another trial showed that a berberis species from India protected the liver from damage by the drug acetaminophen (Gilani and Janbaz, 1992).

Barberry *(Berberis vulgaris)*

The quote found at the beginning of this chapter doesn't come from a modern-day herb conservationist, but from Dr. Harvey Felter in 1922. In his time, goldenseal had already become scarce due to overharvesting in several areas of the country. The situation now, seventy-five years later, is much worse, and barberry as a substitute is just as effective.

Barberry is usually taken as a tincture. For external applications, sores in the mouth, or eye problems, make a tea, and, in the case of the eyes, dilute it. We saw in Chapter 14 that researchers had used berberine successfully to treat eye infections. According to Felter, who was familiar with such treatments, barberry is more effective for this than the isolated berberine alkaloid (Felter and Lloyd, 1898). Traditional uses of barberry include:

blood purifier
chronic diarrhea
dysentery
eye problems
fevers
indigestion
jaundice
laxative
mouth sores and ulcers
tonic

Oregon Grape Root
(Mahonia aquifolium, Berberis aquifolium)

Ellingwood classifies Oregon grape not as a goldenseal substitute, but as an echinacea substitute. He calls it an *antiseptic alterative*. Historically it has been used, like echinacea, for bad blood, although it does not have the excellent reputation that echinacea does for this. It is probably not an immune system stimulant. Felter, on the other hand, did consider it a goldenseal substitute and said of it:

> *Like goldenseal,* Berberis aquifolium *is an excellent peptic bitter and tonic to the gastric function, and is, therefore, a drug of much value in atonic dyspepsia with hepatic torpor. Upon the mucosa its effects are like those of goldenseal, controlling catarrhal outpouring and erosion of tissue.*

(Felter, 1922)

Felter's older medical terminology may be translated to say that Oregon grape is effective in digestive complaints that require a bitter tonic (see Chapter 14), sluggish liver complaints, and chronic mucous membrane problems. If we put these two doctors' opinions together, Oregon grape alone could take the place of the echinacea-goldenseal preparations so common now in health food stores. Oregon grape is especially famous as a treatment for chronic skin conditions.

AN HERBALIST'S TESTIMONY   Northwest herbalist Howie Brounstein has used Oregon grape as a substitute for

BOX 15.1
THE LATIN AND COMMON NAMES
OF OREGON GRAPE

barberry
creeping barberry
mahonia
Mahonia (Berberis) aquifolium
M. nervosa
M. repens
M. pinnata
mountain holly
Odostemon
Oregon grape
Yerba de Sangre

(Source: Moore, 1993)

echinacea and goldenseal, and his experience supports the opinion of the Eclectic physicians that it is a worthy replacement for either. He has used it, for more than ten years, to treat intestinal and other bacterial infections. He often uses it in cases that might otherwise call for a broad-spectrum antibiotic, although he does not consider Oregon grape to be an antibiotic itself. Brounstein recommends taking the tincture in doses of forty-five to sixty drops three or four times a day. If it

is going to work, he says, there should be marked improvement within twenty-four hours. Some of his observations
are recorded in Box 15.2.

BOX 15.2
CONTEMPORARY USE OF OREGON GRAPE AS AN ANTIBIOTIC SUBSTITUTE

ANTIBIOTIC-RESISTANT EAR INFECTIONS:

Every case I have treated has cleared up. I usually add mullein flower oil externally to the ear.

BACTERIAL INFECTION MOVING INWARD:

Excellent results

ABSCESSED TOOTH:

Excellent results

COLDS:

Much better than echinacea for the common
cold. If echinacea is the light cavalry, berberis is
the heavy artillery.

BRONCHITIS:
Good results

BLADDER INFECTIONS:

Mixed results, I generally use other herbs first
and move to berberis in more stubborn cases.

Oregon grape contains a number of alkaloids besides the more famous berberine. Some contemporary herbalists think that these alkaloids may contribute to the sort of broad-spectrum effects that Brounstein notes. Alkaloids found in various species of Oregon grape are:

berberine
berbamine
canadine
jatrorrhizine
mahonine
magnoflorine
oxyacanthine
oxyberberine

Coptis, Gold Thread
(*Coptis chinensis, trifolia*)

In the 1700s and early 1800s in North America, the "King of the Herbs" was gold thread, or *Coptis trifolia*. Says Felter of coptis: "At one time it was so popular as a domestic remedy that more of it was sold in Boston than almost any other remedy" (Felter, 1898). By the early 1800s, it had become overharvested to the point of extinction in the eastern forests west of the Appalachian mountain chain. At about this time, goldenseal was heralded as a substitute for this popular medicinal. Both plants contain the constituent berberine—coptis has even more than goldenseal—and coptis may make a reasonable therapeutic substitute for goldenseal. Coptis contains the alkaloid *coptisine*, which is similar to berberine but is not present in the other plants discussed here. Here is what some early botanical texts say about coptis:

BOX 15.3
THE LATIN AND COMMON NAMES
FOR COPTIS

Anemone groenlandica	canker root
Chrusa borealis	coptide
Coptis chinensis	coptis
C. trifolia	mouth root
Helleborus trifolius	vegetable gold
H. trilobus	yellow root
H. pumilus	

Its use by the colonists was undoubtedly learned from the Native Americans, who used it extensively for mouth sores, poor digestion, and infections. It was used by Mohawks with the sap of White Ash in the ear to treat deafness.

(Erichsen-Brown, 1979)

This plant is one of the rather fine and prompt bitter tonics. It is one of the most grateful appetizers in convalescence from febrile attacks, and in all feeble conditions with weakness of the stomach. It is a popular New England remedy for aphthous sores in the mouth.

(Cook, 1869)

In sore mouth . . . we have repeatedly and promptly cured with the decoction when infusion of hydrastis had no effect. This would seem to indicate that its virtues are not wholly dependent upon berberine. . . . In dyspepsia and in chronic inflammations of the stomach, equal parts of gold-thread and gold-enseal, made into a decoction, with elixir vitriol added in proper quantity, will not only prove effectual, but in many instances of the latter kind, will permanently destroy the appetite for alcoholic beverages.

(Felter and Lloyd, 1898)

Coptis chinensis is an important herb in traditional Chinese medicine, used in that system like the bitter tonics and berberine-containing plants in Western herbalism. Although the trifolia species has made a comeback in American forests since the 1700s, this Chinese species, which is becoming common in the American marketplace, is preferable. It is widely cultivated in China, and harvesting it puts no strain on the ecosystem there. It has a much larger root that *C. trifolia* and contains larger amounts of berberine. Use it in a tincture or tea for the same purposes you would goldenseal or the other herbs named here.

Yerba Mansa *(Anemopsis californica)*

Yerba mansa is a traditional Southwestern herb which is increasingly popular as a goldenseal substitute, primarily on the authority and advice of Southwest herbalist Michael Moore (Moore, 1989). It is one of the most frequently prescribed herbs at our clinic in Boulder, Colorado. Moore, is well-known not only for his scholarship of the herbal scientific literature, but for knowledge of traditional plant use and hands-on knowledge of the plants he writes about. His three volumes are among the most important herbal texts in American history. He didn't come up with the idea of using yerba mansa as a goldenseal substitute out of thin air. You may not have heard of this herb, but don't underrate it because it is not as famous as goldenseal. Traditional residents of the desert areas where it grows consider it among the "royalty" of the local herbs.

Yerba mansa is very different from goldenseal. It contains no berberine or other related alkaloids, and it is not a bitter tonic. It is hot and acrid, with a warming sensation. It may replace goldenseal as a mucous membrane tonic when bitter tonics are contraindicated and the membranes are congested (see Chapter 12).

The Eclectics were aware of Yerba mansa's properties, but generally only those in the western states used it extensively. It was introduced into Eclectic use by Dr. W.H. George of California in 1877—about the same time as echinacea—and remained in use by that profession until its decline in the 1930s. The homeopathic school also used it (Boericke, 1922). The chief Eclectic indication was as a mucous membrane remedy, when there is a full, stuffy sensation in the head and throat, a cough with expectoration, or mucous discharges from the bowels or urinary tract.

CONCLUSION

We've seen that these herbs all either contain constituents in common with goldenseal, or have been used for similar conditions. The Eclectics described several of them as goldenseal substitutes more than seventy-five years ago. I don't personally use them in the place of goldenseal in all conditions, however.

Try this experiment, which I have done. Use some goldenseal and several of its substitutes; I've done this with barberry, Oregon grape root, and yerba mansa, as tinctures. Take a dose, say a dropperful of the tincture or the powdered herb in a little water, and hold it in your mouth. When I take the goldenseal, within a minute I can feel secretions moving in my nasal mucous membranes. In a short time, I can feel stimulation in my intestines and urinary tract membranes. I've never felt this with the goldenseal substitutes, although a combination of Oregon grape root and yerba mansa comes closest.

For this reason, I still use goldenseal when a cold, flu, or bronchitis seems to be going deeper into the system or becoming complicated by a bacterial infection. In one case, a client with a chronic dry bronchitis had been coughing up only slight amounts of clear phlegm for several weeks. Then the discharges turned to yellow and green—a sign of the onset of bacterial infection and the threat of pneumonia. A combination of goldenseal and echinacea returned the phlegm to its normal clear color within twelve hours. Goldenseal is simply the most effective and fastest remedy for

BOX 15.4

THE ECLECTIC APPLICATIONS
OF YERBA MANSA

diarrhea

dysentery

intestinal tonic

mucous membrane tonic

nasal catarrh

respiratory tonic

skin ulcers

tuberculosis

urinary organ tonic

such a condition. I've consulted with two herbalists who were suffering from a similar condition four or five days into a cold. Each of these Southwest herbalists had tried yerba mansa for the condition, without noticeable effect. When they used goldenseal, the got rapid results.

In the following chapters, I'll describe a number of other herbs that may not only act as substitutes for goldenseal and echinacea, but may actually be more effective for specific conditions.

CHAPTER 16

GARLIC

The herbs I have previously described primarily work to strengthen the body's natural defenses against infection rather than attacking microorganisms themselves. Garlic also does this, but with garlic we have a plant that is a true antibiotic. It can effectively kill bacteria, viruses, parasites, fungi, yeasts, and molds, including many that cause serious disease in humans.

GARLIC AS AN ANTIBIOTIC

Garlic is a broad-spectrum antibiotic, killing a wide variety of bacteria. Many pharmaceutical antibiotics kill only a narrow range of these germs. Dr. Tariq Abdullah, a prominent garlic researcher, stated in the August, 1987, issue of *Prevention:* "Garlic has the broadest spectrum of any antimicrobial substance that we know of; it is antibacterial, antifungal, antiparasitic, antiprotozoan, and antiviral." Box 16.1 shows some of the organisms against which researchers have found garlic to be effective. This property belongs to the garlic constituent *allicin*, which is released when you cut a garlic clove. This is the chemical that gives fresh garlic its strong, biting flavor; you need to use fresh garlic to get a reliable antibiotic

BOX 16.1
SOME BACTERIA, VIRUSES, FUNGI, MOLD, AND PARASITES KILLED OR INHIBITED BY GARLIC OR ITS CONSTITUENTS

Acinetobacter calcoaceticus
Aspergillus flavus
Aspergillus fumigatus
Aspergillus parasiticus
Aspergillus niger
Bacillus cereus
Candida albicans
Candida lipolytica
Cryptococcus neoformans
Cryptosporidium
Debaryomyces hansenii
Escherichia coli
Hansenula anomala
Herpes simplex virus type 1
Herpes simplex virus type 2
Histoplasma capsulatum
Human cytomegalovirus (HCMV)
Human immunodeficiency virus (HIV)
Human rhinovirus type 2
Influenza B
Kloeckera apiculata
Lodderomyces elongisporus

Micrococcus luteus

Mycobacterium phlei

Mycobacterium tuberculosis

Paracoccidioides brasiliensis

Parainfluenza virus type 3

Pneumocystis carinii

Proteus vulgaris

Pseudomonas aeruginosa

Rhodotorula rubra

Saccharomyces cerevisiae

Salmonella typhimurium

Salmonella typhimurium

Shigella dysenteriae

Shigella flexneri

Staphylococcus aureus

Streptococcus faecalis

Torulopsis glabrata

Toxoplasma gondii

Vaccinia virus

Vesicular stomatitis virus

Vibrio parahaemolyticus

(Sources: Adetumbi et al, 1983, 1986; Anesini and Perez, 1993; Appleton and Tansey, 1975; Borukh et al, 1974, 1975; Chen et al, 1985; Conner and Beuchat, 1984; Dankert et al, 1979; Didry et al, 1987; Fletcher et al, 1974; Fliermans, 1973; Fromtling and Bulmer, 1978; Ghannoum, 1990; Gonzales-Fandos et al, 1994; Johnson and Vaughn, 1969; Kabelik, 1970; Kumar and Sharma, 1982; Mahajan, 1983; Moore and Atkins, 1977; Sandhu et al, 1980; Sharma et al, 1977; Shashikanth et al, 1984; Tynecka and Gos, 1973, 1975)

effect. Commercial powders and other products will not work for direct applications. Garlic appears to have antibiotic activity whether taken internally or applied topically; researchers found that the urine and blood serum of human subjects taking garlic had activity against fungi (Caporaso et al, 1983).

Resistant Bacteria

A major problem with pharmaceutical antibiotics is that they can promote the development of resistant strains of bacteria. Initially the antibiotic kills most of the bacteria being attacked. With repeated exposure, however, those few bacteria that by chance are genetically resistant to the antibiotic begin to multiply. Eventually, a recurring infection becomes completely resistant to that antibiotic. After a half-century of the massive use of antibiotics, and the indiscriminate over-prescription of them in North America, potentially serious medical problems exist from resistant strains of bacteria. Garlic does not seem to produce such resistant strains, and may be effective against strains that have become resistant to pharmaceutical antibiotics.

European researchers in the late 1970s tested garlic juice against a group of ten different bacteria and yeasts (Moore and Atkins, 1977). They found that garlic was effective against all of them, and also found a "complete absence of development of resistance." In an East Indian study of garlic used to treat dysentery, the researchers specifically selected four bacterial strains that were resistant to multiple antibiotics (Chowdhury et al, 1991).

Garlic is effective against specific bacteria that are notorious for developing resistant strains, such as staphylococcus, mycobacterium, salmonella, and species of proteus.

ANTIVIRAL ACTIVITY

A weakness of conventional antibiotics is that they are not effective against viral infections. That's why they won't work against the common cold or flu. They also won't work against such serious viral infections as viral meningitis, viral pneumonia, or herpes infections. Garlic or its constituents will directly kill influenza, herpes, vaccinia (cowpox), vesicular stomatitis virus (responsible for cold sores), and human cytomegalovirus (a common source of secondary infection in AIDS). Garlic will also cure or improve the symptoms from a variety of viral diseases in humans or animals. In one animal study, researchers first fed a garlic extract to mice. They then introduced the flu virus into the nasal passages of the animals. Those animals that had received the garlic were protected from the flu, while the untreated animals all got sick. The researchers postulated that garlic's effect was due in part to direct antiviral effects of garlic, and in part to stimulation of the immune system (Adetumbi and Lau, 1983).

PARASITES AND FUNGI

The medical missionary Albert Schweitzer brought some fame to garlic earlier this century when he used it successfully to treat amoebic dysentery in his patients in equatorial Africa. Subsequent experiments have shown garlic to be effective not only against the parasitic amoebas that cause dysentery, but against other organisms such as toxoplasma, cryptosporidia, and pneumocystis, all of which cause disease in humans.

Parasitic infections are a common problem in AIDS patients. Dr. Subhuti Dharmananda, director of the Immune Enhancement Project in Portland, Oregon, regularly treats

AIDS patients who have such opportunistic infections. The main antibiotic therapy he uses is garlic, at about nine cloves a day for active infections. He finds it effective in preventing or treating these infections, even when conventional antibiotics have failed to do so. Note that he started out trying to use an encapsulated form of garlic standardized for its allicin content—one of the better products. He found, however, that even doses of twenty-seven capsules a day had no effect on the infections. When he switched to raw garlic at the same dose, he got the desired result (Dharmananda, 1995). Recent research supports use for intestinal parasites in AIDS (AIDS Research Alliance, 1996; Deshpande et al, 1993).

YEAST INFECTIONS

If you've ever had athlete's foot, you know how stubborn a yeast or fungal infection can be. A garlic wash can be very effective against fungi externally, but garlic can also treat systemic fungal infections. Researchers from the University of New Mexico demonstrated that garlic was effective both in the test tube and in animals against infection with the fungus *Cryptococcus neoformans* (Fromtling and Bulmer, 1978). Chinese researchers also have shown that garlic as an intravenous extract can be effective against cryptococcal meningitis. The blood and cerebrospinal fluid of the patients in that trial was twice as effective against the fungus as before treatment with garlic (Davis et al., 1990).

HOW TO USE GARLIC

To use garlic as an antibiotic, take it internally and, if appropriate, apply it directly to an infection. For internal use, try one of the following forms:

- Garlic-infused wine: Chop or crush garlic, cover with wine, and let it sit overnight.
- Garlic vinegar: Same as above, but use vinegar instead of wine.
- Garlic honey: Same as above, but use honey. No added water is needed. This makes a great antibiotic cough syrup.
- Garlic/carrot juice: Blend three cloves of garlic in six ounces of carrot juice; let it sit for four to six hours.

For external application, use caution putting crushed garlic directly against the skin, because it can cause burns. Here are some forms you can use for direct application of garlic as an antibiotic:

- Blend three cloves of garlic in a quart of water and apply as a wash. Make a larger amount of this mixture and use it as a foot bath for infections of the feet or as a sitz bath for the pelvic area.
- Crush garlic and dilute the juice with ten parts of water. Use it as nose drops or a gargle.

GARLIC AND THE IMMUNE SYSTEM

Although garlic attacks bacteria, viruses, and other microorganisms directly, it also stimulates the body's natural defenses against these invaders. Garlic's remarkable and legendary power against infectious diseases is due to a combination of both of these properties.

Garlic or its constituents activate phagocytes, B-cells, and T-cells—all three levels of the cellular immune system. For instance, diallyl trisulfide, a constituent of garlic, was found to activate natural killer cells and macrophages directly, and to indirectly increase B-cell activity to make antibodies. It did this in lab experiments at concentrations of as low as one microgram per milliliter—the equivalent of a tiny pinch of salt in thirty gallons of water. The macrophages in this trial were then tested for their activity against cancer cells, and the diallyl-trisulfide-treated cells were more active than regular macrophages, indicating that not only their number but their activity was increased (Feng et al, 1994). This same effect has been reproduced in other experiments.

This effect is not limited to trials in a test tube. Dr. Abdullah experimented with garlic to treat AIDS, giving the equivalent of two cloves of garlic a day to ten patients for six weeks, and the equivalent of four cloves for another six weeks. Three of the patients could not complete the trial, but of the seven who did, all showed normal natural killer cell activity by the end of the trial—activity which had been depressed at the start of the trial. The patients' opportunistic infections—chronic diarrhea, candida infection, genital herpes, and a chronic sinus infection—all diminished. The patient with the chronic sinus infection had gained no relief from antibiotics during more than a year of treatment before the garlic trial (Abdullah, 1989).

In one trial, immune system parameters of the blood were measured after elderly patients took a garlic powder preparation for three months (Brosche and Platt, 1993, 1994). The dose was only 600 mg of the powder per day, the equivalent of less than one-third of a garlic clove. Blood tests showed an increase in phagocytosis of the white blood cells, and also increased numbers of lymphocytes, responsible for cell-mediated immunity. Other trials have shown that garlic can increase the activity of natural killer cells in healthy volunteers (Kandil et al, 1987, 1988).

TABLE 16.1   SOME CONDITIONS THAT
CAN BE EFFECTIVELY
TREATED WITH GARLIC

(Note: Crushed garlic applied directly to the skin can cause burns.)

Bites and Stings	Apply crushed and moistened garlic directly to the bite or sting
Bronchitis	Use raw garlic in one of the forms listed above
Candida infection	Use both internal and external applications if appropriate
Common Cold	Take internally
Diarrhea and Dysentery	Take internally
Ear Infections	Soak crushed garlic in oil, and apply the oil directly to the ear
Fungal Infections	Apply garlic oil directly or blend garlic in warm water to make a soak or compress; also take internally
Herpes	Take fresh garlic orally, and apply garlic blended in a little water directly to the sore
Infections	Take garlic internally and apply directly to an infected wound
Influenza	Take internally at the first threat of exposure
Parasites	Blend three cloves in a palatable medium and take internally, three times a day, for a total of nine cloves
Vaginal Infection	Use a douche, with three garlic cloves blended in a quart of water; strain through cheesecloth first to remove the solid matter

A CONNOISSEUR'S GARLIC COCKTAIL

Different solvents extract and promote specific chemical reactions between the constituents of garlic. Water, vinegar, alcohol, and oil each draw specific constituents out. Alcohol and water together, for instance, make the best solvent for extracting allicin. Soaking crushed garlic in oil promotes the production of ajoenes and dithiins, important antibiotic and blood-thinning constituents of garlic. My garlic "cocktail," then, is as follows:

> 3 cloves of garlic
> 1 tablespoon of red wine
> 1 tablespoon of vinegar
> 1 tablespoon of olive oil

Blend well in a blender. Add 1/4 cup hot water. Let stand for six hours. Do not strain. Add one-third of this mixture to a cup of hot water. Repeat every three to six hours until the cocktail is all gone.

On paper, this sounds a little like drinking salad dressing, but I find it to be a pleasant, stimulating tonic with a sharp taste. Raw garlic cloves upset my intestines, but this does not.

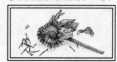

CHAPTER 17

HERBS FOR COLD AND FLU

Echinacea and goldenseal are probably used most often in this country for colds and flu. Echinacea is certainly helpful for those conditions, but goldenseal is almost entirely wasted in acute infections. There are several other herbs, however, that are much more potent in these conditions. Osha, like echinacea, works best at the onset of infection. Two other herbs, boneset and elderberry, are much more potent to knock the cold out quickly. These two herbs should be in the medicine cabinet of everyone who is particularly at risk from influenza. We saw in Chapter 16 that fresh garlic (not garlic pills) is also a good preventive.

ECHINACEA

Echinacea has the remarkable ability to abort a cold or flu if you catch it early enough. Up to a teaspoon of the tincture taken every two or three hours will usually keep the cold at bay. Once the cold or flu is well established, however, echinacea is not the best single herb to use, although it is useful

237

in combinations. It may shorten the duration or severity of the infection, and even save lives in the frail elderly, but won't usually "knock out" the cold.

The Schöneberger clinical trial I cited in Chapter 6 showed that echinacea could prevent colds in people who are especially susceptible to them. The results were less than spectacular in shortening the duration or severity of a cold, however. The average length of the colds in individuals who took echinacea was still five to seven days—hardly helpful to get you back to work. The Bräunig trial also showed that an echinacea tincture could shorten the duration of a cold, but again, differences from the placebo group were not very dramatic at the four-day measurements.

The Eclectics did not consider echinacea to be a major remedy for the flu, preferring remedies such as boneset. Felter says that epidemic influenza is only "occasionally" ameliorated by echinacea, although he favors it as an auxiliary herb (Felter, 1898, 1922). Ellingwood also mentions it, but only as an auxiliary herb.

The widespread use of echinacea to treat colds and flu in this country is based more on its widespread fame—and on the lack of knowledge by the general public of these more effective remedies—than on the best clinical indications.

BONESET (EUPATORIUM PERFOLIATUM)

Boneset is one of the first North American herbs to be learned of from the Native Americans; its use was taught to the Pilgrims as a flu remedy. In parts of the colonies, flu was called "breakbone fever" which described the aches and pains associated with the condition. Boneset got its name as a treatment for the fever, not because it has any effect on the bones.

It was exported to England for that use by the end of the 1600s. In the nineteenth century, it was one of the few herbs used by all schools of medicine and herbalism—Eclectic, Thompsonian, Physiomedicalist, Homeopathic, and Allopathic—and was known as *the* remedy for flu. It was also recognized as a panacea for both chronic and acute illnesses by the Native, Anglo, and African-American cultures. African-American slaves in the South used it to treat fevers and as a general tonic. It is a mystery of medical history that such a potent medicine could descend from being a domestic panacea to being completely left out of some modern herbals. Some possible properties than would inhibit its popularity are its bitter flavor and its ability to cause nausea in larger doses. In one modern textbook of medical botany, the authors include boneset in their chapter on famous herbal panaceas:

> *Extolled for its many properties and uses against intermittent fevers, arthritis, gout, and epilepsy by early American physicians and Native Americans,* E. perfoliatum *was a virtual panacea and was always found in the well-regulated household. It was widely used by Confederate troops, who drank hot infusions of the plant as a febrifuge [fever-reducer] and as a substitute for quinine.*

(Lewis and Elvin-Lewis, 1977)

Don't confuse the plant with *Eupatorium purpureum*, usually known as Queen-of-the-meadow, but sometimes called "purple boneset." *E. purpureum* is primarily used as a diuretic. The use of both plants was taught to New England colonists by Native American herbalist Joe Pye, but his name stuck only to *E. purpureum,* which is sometimes called "Joe Pye weed."

Boneset has had a dual role in the history of American herbalism, being equally valuable in treating acute and chronic conditions. It was used in cold infusion for chronic conditions, and hot infusion for acute conditions. Most people think of it now as a fever-lowering flu remedy, but part of its historical panacea status was its use as a tonic in chronic disease.

A recent article in my *Medical Herbalism* newsletter contains a letter about boneset from herbalist Sasha Daucus of Doniphan, Missouri:

> At our clinic, a nursing-based wellness practice, I use boneset as a first line of defense if I suspect a viral rather than a bacterial infection. I use ten drops of the tincture in hot water, every half hour for up to five doses, to encourage sweating. For ongoing flu symptoms (or herpes) I use ten drops four times daily. If taken at the first signs of flu or herpes, very often neither condition will express. If used later in the course of a flu, many cases will clear up quickly. It should be taken no more than five days running, which is seldom necessary: I advise clients that if it's working, they'll feel better after the first day or two at most.

> ## CASE STUDY
>
> The most recent case was a thirty-eight-year-old woman, a registered nurse, who came to the clinic

after having been unable to work for nearly two weeks. The symptoms had begun with nausea and vomiting and extreme fatigue. At the point when I saw her, she was past the acute stage but was still seriously fatigued and had a poor appetite. She had been prescribed antibiotics by an M.D., which she had taken for the full ten-day course with no sign of improvement. I recommended ten drops of boneset immediately, and then four times daily for five days. I expected she would feel significantly better after a few doses, and told her to call me the next day to check in. When she did, she was delighted. She said: "After the first dose, I felt normal for the first time since I got this. I'd been feeling 'unreal,' like I was isolated from the world behind some kind of wall. That's gone and I feel like I've returned to myself again."

(Daucus, 1995)

Echinacea is used in combination with boneset in many German products, and physicians often use it instead of echinacea to treat the flu (Weiss, 1988). A German clinical study performed in 1987 showed that a combination of echinacea and boneset was effective for treating colds and flu (Amman and Suter, 1987). Weiss says that the echinacea-boneset combination is indicated above all in acute viral infections when antibiotics are ineffective.

The immune-system-stimulating polysaccharides in boneset were found to be ten times more potent than echinacea polysaccharides in one study (Wagner and Proksch,

1985), and immune-system-stimulating sesquiterpene lactones have also been identified (Wren, 1989). The Eclectics found that boneset has a strong influence on the lungs, and helps relieve coughs (Cook, 1869; Felter and Lloyd, 1898).

The Proper Use of Boneset

The dried flowering tops [leaves and flowers] of boneset are used for medicine. The drying may be important. The fresh plant contains a toxic constituent, tremetrol, which is greatly reduced by drying. This is not the plant to use for making a fresh plant tincture. When milking animals eat the fresh plant, the tremetrol in their milk can cause "milk sickness" in humans, with symptoms such as nausea, vomiting, appetite loss, thirst, and constipation (Willard, 1991).

An old herbal text states that, in the early 1800s, boneset was found hanging to dry in "every household or barn." I suggest that you keep some in yours.

BONESET TEA   As a hot infusion, boneset was traditionally used to induce sweating and/or vomiting. A standard hot infusion is an ounce of the herb in a quart of boiling water; cover and let cool a bit. This is not one to take by the cupful; the dose is one to three ounces, or less than half a teacup. Cook says to repeat the dose "until the desired objects are obtained," which means sweat or vomit. Induced vomiting as a therapy has almost passed completely out of Western herbalism and medicine, and boneset's ability to cause vomiting may have helped to kill the plant's reputation. Those properties are easy to avoid by sticking to low doses.

BLACK ELDER *(SAMBUCUS NIGRA)*

Black elder is another famous flu remedy from traditional medicine; its recorded medical uses go back to at least the time of the Romans. A recent clinical trial performed in Israel showed that a preparation not only ended cases of the flu within three days, but also boosted the immune system. Although this herb is not nearly as well researched as echinacea, it also appears to have immune-system-stimulating properties. Some of the traditional medical uses of black elder are:

alterative
blood purifier
bronchitis
chronic skin ulcers
colds
eczema
erysipelas
flu
nasal catarrh
rheumatoid arthritis
sciatica
sore throats
syphilis

Elderberry Teas

The elderberry flowers have traditionally been used to make teas to treat colds and sore throats; taken hot before bed, a cup will usually induce perspiration. British herbal authority Maude Grieve says:

Refreshing sleep will follow, and the patient will
wake up well on the way to recovery and the cold
or influenza will probably be banished within thirty-
six hours.

(Grieve, 1930)

The tea, taken cold daily, was historically considered
a spring medicine and a blood purifier. In earlier times, before the advent of refrigerators, transportation, and the in-
dustrialization of food, people's diets changed radically
between summer and winter. In winter, they ate mainly
meat and stored grains without fresh fruits or vegetables.
Life also tended to become more sedentary during the
cold weather, with farm work at a low ebb. Thus, by spring-
time people were sluggish and toxic from the heavy diet
and were more prone to illness. Spring tonics, or blood
cleansers, were a common traditional remedy in such soci-
eties. Black elder was such a tonic in nineteenth-century
Britain. Contemporary German physician R.F. Weiss attests
to this "spring tonic" action and says that "the resistance-
enhancing action does indeed come into play." He lists the
plant in his medical textbook as a treatment for colds and flu
(Weiss, 1988).

Elderberry was an official medicine listed in the *U.S.*
Pharmacopoeia from the year of its founding in 1820 until
1890 when, along with many other herbal remedies, it was
dropped (Boyle, 1991). In North American naturopathic
medicine, it has been used as a blood purifier. A naturopathic
textbook from the 1950s says that the cold infusion "is an excellent alterative and diuretic in many dermal manifestations
of metabolic toxicosis." This, translated, means that it will

assist an overloaded immune system. The naturopaths used it both internally and externally for eczema, and applied it externally to "indolent ulcers" and persistent skin inflammations (Kuts-Chereaux, 1953).

Elderberry Juice

From these traditional indications, it is clear that black elder, among other things, builds up the resistance of the immune system. Recent research performed in Israel and Panama has demonstrated that the juice from the berries of this plant not only stimulates the immune system, but also directly inhibits the influenza virus (Zakay-Rones et al, 1995; Mumcuoglu, 1995). The juice of the berries, made into a syrup, is another traditional form of use for the black elder plant. It has less tendency to induce sweating, but is considered effective in most of the same conditions as the tea of the flowers (Grieve, 1930).

Israeli researcher Madeleine Mumcuoglu, Ph.D., of the Hadassah-Hebrew University Medical Center in Ein Karem, Israel, performed the initial research, and found that juice seems to be designed as a specific weapon against the flu virus. The influenza virus forms tiny spikes, called *hemagglutinins*, which are laced with an enzyme called *neuraminidase*. This enzyme helps the virus to penetrate the cell walls of a healthy organism. The virus then sets up shop in the cell, reproducing more cell-busting viruses. The active ingredients that Mumcuoglu discovered disarm the neuraminidase enzyme within twenty-four to forty-eight hours, halting the spread of the virus.

In clinical trials, patients who took the elderberry juice syrup reported fast termination of symptoms. Twenty percent reported significant improvement within twenty-four hours, and seventy percent in forty-eight hours; ninety percent claimed a complete cure after three days. Patients receiving the placebo required six days for recovery. As proof that black elder has more in it than the enzyme-neutralizing constituents, researchers found that the patients who took it also had higher levels of antibodies against the flu virus.

Treatment for Mutating Flu

Elderberry has been proven effective against eight different influenza viruses. This may solve the perennial problem of the "mutating flu." Viruses have the ability to alter their genes and create new strains. This makes a problem for creating vaccines against viral diseases, such as flu or AIDS, because the vaccine can only be developed against known strains. The host remains unprotected against newly evolved forms of the virus. With the flu virus, the new evolving forms can sometimes be quite deadly.

Periodically, especially deadly strains of flu develop. We haven't had an outbreak of deadly flu in recent decades, so many people do not realize how serious the illness can be. One strain killed more than 21,000,000 people worldwide in the second decade of this century—that's more than died in World War I. Some epidemiologists have pointed out in recent years that we are overdue for another deadly flu epidemic, which reoccur, like earthquakes, at regular but not necessarily predictable intervals. Vaccines will be of no use against a new strain, at least when it initially appears.

Black elder may thus be able to literally save lives, because most strains of the virus use the same enzyme mechanism to penetrate cells. Black elder preparations may be superior to flu shots for another reason: fifty percent of people who get the vaccines report side effects (Zakay-Rones, 1995; Mumcuoglu, 1995).

The beneficial constituents of black elder are not soluble in alcohol, so use the tea or the juice rather than the tincture. A syrup of the juice—the same one used in the Israeli clinical trial—is available in health food stores as Sambucol. Be sure to use preparations of black elder *(Sambuca nigra)* rather than the common elder species, several of which are poisonous.

OSHA *(LIGUSTICUM PORTERI)*

Osha was, to the native inhabitants of the high altitudes of the Rocky Mountains, what echinacea was to the natives of the Great Plains—their most important plant for treating infections. It is one of the most-often-prescribed plants by herbalists in that region today, including those at our clinic at the Rocky Mountain Center for Botanical Studies in Boulder, Colorado. We use osha extensively to treat colds, flu, sore throats, and bronchial infections. The tincture or tea is antibacterial and can be used as a wash or compress on cuts, abrasions, infected wounds, ulcers, or herpes sores. It is also a potent antiviral herb. In the petri dish, its constituent *Z-ligustilide* is about half as potent as ribavirin (Virazole), a conventional antiviral drug used against viruses such as influenza and herpes (Beck and Stermitz, 1995).

The antiviral constituents of osha are soluble only in alcohol, so you will need to chew the dried root—the traditional method—take dried capsules, or use a tincture. If you use the capsules, break them open and put them in some

TABLE 17.1   HERBS TO USE DURING VARIOUS
STAGES OF A COLD

Stage	Application	Herbs
Prevention	Use during cold season if you are particularly susceptible to catching cold	echinacea, garlic, astragalus, reishi
Epidemics	Use when a flu is "going around" or when you have been exposed; use smaller doses	echinacea, garlic osha, boneset, elderberry juice
First onset	Use when you feel the first symptoms coming on	echinacea (large doses), osha (large doses), boneset, elderberry juice or tea
Full-blown	Use when a cold or flu is solidly established	boneset, elderberry juice or tea, echinacea (smaller doses, repeated every two hours)
Complicated	Use when complications, such as bacterial infections, appear or the cold suddenly seems to go "deeper" into the system	boneset and elderberry are especially important; if mucus has stopped flowing freely and mucous membranes are infected, or if green or yellow mucous begins to appear, use goldenseal
Lingering	When low-grade symptoms persist after the otherwise normal course of the cold	boneset, elderberry, echinacea, or, if mucous membranes are involved, goldenseal

warm water so that the membranes of your mouth and throat can be exposed to the herb. For colds and flu it works best, like echinacea, if you take it at the first signs of infection. Use it in higher doses—up to a teaspoon of the tincture every two or three hours—to abort a cold.

Southwest herbalist Michael Moore, who has taught the use of this plant widely and introduced the larger herbal community to it, tells how to make an osha cough syrup:

> *Grind up the root, and steep in twice its volume of honey over low heat for an hour, then press out [the plant material] when it is partially cooled.*
>
> (Moore, 1979)

A similar plant *(Ligusticum wallichi)* is used in Chinese medicine to induce uterine contractions, so osha is probably contraindicated in pregnancy.

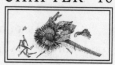

CHAPTER 18

HERBS THAT PROMOTE GENERAL RESISTANCE

The herbs I've described so far are ones you can take when you're getting sick or are already sick. In this chapter, I'll describe some herbs you can take when you are not ill if your immunity is generally run down and you want to prevent illness. Refer to Chapter 10 for lifestyle modifications that will also build up your general resistance.

Many of these herbs are superior to echinacea for prevention, rather than treatment, of illnesses. Some are classified as *adaptogens*—plants that increase your ability to respond to any form of stress. They are all used in traditional Asian medicine. Several of them, or constituents isolated from them, are used by conventional physicians today in China, Japan, and the U.S. to treat cancer, AIDS, and autoimmune diseases.

The Asian herbs are now beginning to appear in health food stores in a variety of forms. Some appear as alcohol tinctures, which is not the way the Asians use them, and not the way I recommend. They should be made into teas or tonic "soups," or eaten as foods the way the Asians consume them.

ASTRAGALUS
(*ASTRAGALUS MEMBRANACEUS*)

Astragalus is an herb from traditional Chinese medicine that has been successfully transplanted to North American herbal practice. In a survey of the top fifty herbs used by clinical herbalists in the U.S., astragalus placed sixteenth. It is one of the best herbs worldwide for building resistance to colds and infections. It also figures prominently in the herbal treatment of cancer, AIDS, and autoimmune diseases. It builds overall immunity, strengthens the lungs, and improves the digestion. It increases endurance and body weight in animals. American varieties of astragalus are known as "locoweed" because of their overstimulating effects on cattle that eat too much of them.

In Chinese medical terms, astragalus builds up the *protective chi*. Imagine that there is a protective shield around your body, just below the surface of the skin, that keeps out cold and other external influences. It vitalizes the non-specific immune system defenses and wards off infections. This is the protective chi, and astragalus is the premier herb in Chinese herbalism for strengthening it.

Astragalus, in combination with another tonic herb, ligustrum, gained fame as a possible immune-system-stimulating and anti-cancer herb in scientific circles in the 1980s. In one trial with nineteen cancer patients, water extracts of astragalus restored the function of the T-cells in ninety percent of the patients. In another trial, these two herbs in a broader formula increased the survival time of cancer patients receiving chemotherapy. Formulas based on these two herbs are used today in AIDS clinics at the Institute for Traditional Medicine in Portland, Oregon, and the Qwan Yin Clinic in San Francisco.

Astragalus is a warming herb, and is especially beneficial when cool or cold weather comes on, or if you work or play for long periods outdoors and are exposed to cold wind. It has no known toxicity, but can cause discomfort if you have a tendency to feel hot. It is available as a long, yellow-colored sliced root that looks something like a tongue depressor. It is also widely available in health food stores as encapsulated powders, teas, and tinctures. I recommend that you buy the whole root and make your own tea. Simmer it in a pot of water for a half hour, or add it to soups. Remove the root from the soup before eating.

GINSENG

Asian Ginseng *(Panax ginseng)*

Asian ginseng is one of the most famous herbs worldwide, and in Chinese medicine it is the king of the tonic herbs. It is one of the most potent adaptogens we have. It is unparalleled for building up your energy if you are depleted. It has to be taken with care, however, because it can be overstimulating, causing insomnia, tension, and discomfort. Most Americans who feel "wiped out" will find American or Siberian ginsengs more suitable for their constitutions.

Asian ginseng is not specifically an immune system stimulant, but greatly improves your ability to handle stresses of any sort, and thus helps you to adapt to the conditions that might promote illness. There are many forms of ginseng available in health food stores, drug stores, and supermarkets. Many of these products have so little ginseng in them that they won't do you much good. See my book, *The Healing Power of Ginseng,* for a detailed description of products and forms. I recommend that you either buy the whole root and make a tea, or purchase a product from one of the companies listed in Appendix B. Take ginseng for six to eight weeks at a time, and then take a two-week break.

American Ginseng
(Panax quinquefolium)

Although American and Asian ginseng share the same name, they are quite different in their overall effects on the system. Whereas Asian ginseng is considered warming in traditional Chinese medical terms, American ginseng is cooling. Asian ginseng is usually contraindicated during summer weather or when you are hot and sweating from other causes, but American ginseng is perfect for this. It can help cool, calm, moisten, and strengthen a run-down system. It is very well suited to stressed, overworked, and overactive Americans. It also specifically strengthens the lungs. It has to be taken for three to six weeks to get its full benefit. American ginseng is quite expensive, and products are of variable quality in the U.S. marketplace. You might find the other herbs in this section gentler on your pocketbook.

Siberian Ginseng, Eleuthero Root
(*Eleutherococcus senticosus*)

Siberian ginseng is not really "ginseng" at all. That name was added to it by American marketing companies hoping to capitalize on the popularity of ginseng. It was researched and perfected as a medicine by Russian researchers. A large volume of research shows that it is an excellent adaptogen without as much tendency to overstimulate as Asian ginseng, although when overused it can cause tension and insomnia. It also has more immediate tonic effects than ginseng. It is widely used today in Russia to increase resistance to stress, colds, and flu, and is very effective for those purposes.

The Siberian ginseng products in the North American marketplace are generally of poor quality. A Canadian regulatory commission examined three lots of this herb coming into that country from Asia, and found that two of them contained herbs other than eleutherococcus, and that the other lot was five percent caffeine. The Russian product that was so extensively researched is highly concentrated, with one part of the herb to each part of solvent, extracted in thirty-three percent alcohol. Many American products use only one part of the herb to five parts of a solvent with much higher alcohol content. The two forms are not equivalent. The only company I am aware of that markets a product made to the Russian specifications is HerbPharm in Williams, Oregon. They then use vacuum concentration to make it double strength. If you want the same benefits that the Russians receive from eleuthero root during their long winter, I suggest that you use the same preparation that they do.

LICORICE ROOT (*GLYCYRRHIZA GLABRA*)

Licorice is famous in the West as a candy, but most licorice candy is made from anise flavorings, rather than from real licorice. This herb is much more than a candy, however. It is in the same general category of herbs as ginseng in Chinese medicine. It is probably the most versatile herb in either Eastern or Western pharmacopoeias, and can benefit respiratory illnesses, digestive problems, menstrual disorders, inflammatory conditions, autoimmune diseases, and chronic liver disease. Its chief benefit for building the resistance is that it can enhance the function of the adrenal glands, helping to cope with many forms of stress.

Licorice root can cause side effects when taken in large doses and for long periods. It stimulates the adrenal glands and adds to the effect of steroid hormones; the effect is to cause high blood pressure, edema, headache, and potassium loss. These effects were first observed in people who ate large amounts of concentrated licorice extracts in candy. Later they were observed in the long-term clinical use of licorice for the treatment of ulcers and hepatitis. They do not appear with normal use, but if you have a tendency to high blood pressure and edema, try another of the herbs named here.

You can make a licorice infusion or decoction by itself, or add licorice to your other teas. See Appendix A for directions.

GANODERMA, REISHI
(*GANODERMA LUCIDUM*)

The ganoderma mushroom, sometimes called by the Japanese name *reishi* in the U.S., is an immune-system-stimulating sedative. It is one of the prized medicines in traditional Chinese medicine. A large amount of scientific research has been conducted into ganoderma, especially in Japan. It builds resistance to infection and tumors, and has cardiotonic properties, lowering serum cholesterol and increasing blood circulation through the coronary arteries. It is my personal favorite herb for treating autoimmune diseases. A number of clinical trials have shown it to be effective in treating chronic bronchitis. Ganoderma is especially useful as a sedative for the nervousness, restlessness, and insomnia that often accompany general deficiency.

There are two types of ganoderma available in the U.S. as whole dried mushrooms. A red one is round and dense, with a slightly bitter flavor. The black one is larger and more fibrous or fleshy, and tastes salty. The one you want is the red one. Get the whole dried mushrooms, make a decoction, and drink it daily during times of weakness or stress. Follow the instructions in Appendix A, but decoct the mushrooms on low heat for two to three hours.

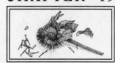

CHAPTER 19

OTHER
USEFUL
WESTERN
HERBS

In previous chapters, I've only begun to touch on the herbs that may be useful in treating infections or chronic immune system weakness. In this chapter, I'll describe some of the most important blood purifiers, lymphatic herbs, antibiotics, and antiparasitic herbs.

BLOOD PURIFIERS

I described "blood purifiers" in Chapter 3, when explaining the Eclectic use of echinacea. Several herbs discussed in Chapter 17 are also blood purifiers. The berberine-containing herbs described in Chapter 15 are also blood purifiers. The following are two more herbs from that category. These are both well-suited to the less serious conditions listed in Box 3.2.

Burdock *(Arctium lappa)*

Burdock ranked eleventh in a recent poll of U.S. medical herbalists' most important herbs (Bergner, 1994). It ranks in my personal top three for frequency of prescription to my patients. No scientific research exists into burdock or its constituents, but it has been important in Western traditional medicine for thousands of years. Burdock enhances liver function by promoting the flow of bile; it also increases blood circulation to the skin, and is a mild diuretic.

The Eclectics considered burdock a lymphatic herb, promoting the flow of lymph. The homeopath Hale even stated that it was equivalent in its lymphatic action to poke root, a toxic herb used for serious lymphatic congestion and tumors. Burdock is also a traditional anti-cancer herb, appearing in a number of formulas used in the last century to treat cancer. It is my number-one herb for treating boils. Burdock contains high amounts of *inulin*, which may have an effect on the immune system. Other inulin-containing plants, such as dandelion root and elecampagne, are widely used as blood purifiers or tonics.

Take burdock root as a decoction (see Appendix A), in normal beverage quantities, up to four cups a day. You don't have to be sick to take burdock as a beverage. Its properties will help keep you well, and it makes an excellent coffee substitute.

Cleavers *(Galium aparine)*

Cleavers is another herb for which little scientific research exists. Like burdock, however, it has a strong reputation among traditional herbalists as a blood purifier and lymphatic herb. It is used today as a cooling remedy in treating fevers and inflammations, and for treating swollen glands and urinary tract infections. Its lymph-promoting properties are partly responsible for its "blood purifying" effects. As we saw in Chapter 4, an increased flow of lymph promotes enhanced circulation of the immune system weapons of the lymph glands, including T-cells and antibodies. It may also purify the blood through its diuretic properties.

LYMPHATIC HERBS

Both of the herbs described above have reputations as lymph-promoting herbs, but they are used for broader indications as well. The two herbs that follow are more specific to the lymphatic system, and may be used for acutely swollen glands.

Red Root *(Ceanothus spp.)*

The Eclectics used red root for stagnancy of the *portal venous system*. The is the series of veins that carries nutrients from the digestive tract to the liver for processing before it can enter the general circulation. Like other venous blood, portal blood has no pulse or pressure. It also has to move upward, against gravity, to get to the liver. A sedentary lifestyle, a heavy diet, intestinal disorders, and liver stagnancy can all cause this network to become stagnant. This affects immunity because blood from the spleen, a lymphatic organ that filters the blood, must also drain through the portal system. Key Eclectic indications for the use of red root were a swollen spleen and a stagnant liver. It was used by soldiers during the Civil War for spleen inflammations that accompany malaria.

Portal venous stagnation is invariably accompanied by stagnation of lymph. About two-thirds of the lymph in the body is derived from the portal system. The lymph from most of the body passes through the same anatomical area as the venous blood on its way back to the general circulation near the heart, and is pumped by the same mechanisms. Thus, red root is also considered a lymphatic herb. We don't know exactly how it works, but red root is clinically effective not only for enlarged spleen, but for such lymphatic conditions as swollen glands, pelvic congestion, and ovarian cysts.

According to herbalist Michael Moore, the dose for the tincture is large: one-half to one-and-one-half teaspoons three or four times a day. The dose for the tea is small, however, from one-eighth to one-quarter cup of a standard decoction (see Appendix A). He also recommends a milder tea in larger quantities: two tablespoons of the root boiled for twenty minutes in a quart of water; take a third of the quart an hour before each meal.

Note that the very best mover of portal venous blood and lymph is aerobic exercise. The vigorous deep breathing and pumping of the diaphragm mechanically move the blood and lymph out of the abdomen and into the general circulation. A high-fat diet promotes lymphatic stagnancy as well, because all the fats from the digestive system must be drained through the lymphatic vessels before they reach the general circulation. More fat makes for "thicker" lymph after meals.

Ocotillo (Fouquieria splendens)

According to herbalist Michael Moore, this Southwestern plant is a specific for lymphatic and venous congestions of the pelvic area. This could include conditions ranging from swollen pelvic glands to hemorrhoids, to uterine fibroids. This is not a well-known plant, and may not be available in some health food stores, but we use it consistently in our clinic for conditions of pelvic congestion. The dose is two droppers of the tincture four times a day.

Antibiotics

The following herbs, unlike most I've described so far, are true antibiotics. Usnea will kill germs, molds, fungi, and other microorganisms when applied topically, but will also treat such conditions as bronchitis, pneumonia, or urinary tract infections. A constituent in uva ursi breaks down to produce an antibiotic substance in the body which is then excreted in the urine, delivering the antibiotic directly to the urinary tract.

Usnea, Old Man's Beard *(Usnea spp.)*

Usnea species are antibiotic and antifungal lichens that hang like little beards from trees throughout the forests of the Pacific Northwest. Thus its traditional name, "old man's beard." A lichen is not really a plant, but a fungus and algae living together as a single organism. The fungus provides a rigid structure for the chlorophyll-rich algae, which cover the fungus and provide nutrition for both. Together they produce constituents different from those of either original organism—chemicals with unique antibiotic and antifungal properties to protect the lichen from microorganisms. These compounds are useful for their antibiotic effects in humans as well, especially for urinary and respiratory tract infections, athlete's foot, and other fungal infections. Usnea ointments are common medicinal agents in Europe, used for topical fungal infections.

Usnea appears to have immune-system-enhancing properties as well. European preparations have been shown to enhance resistance to colds and flu (Weiss, 1988). *Alectoria usneoides*, a close relative that is often found hanging from the same tree as usnea, was used in traditional Arabian medicine for a swollen spleen, another possible indication that it affects the immune system favorably. Related species *(Usnea diffticata, longissima)* are used in traditional Chinese medicine to treat respiratory infections and skin ulcers. Usnea has been used in traditional European medicine for mucous membrane infections, diarrhea, dysentery, and weakness of the stomach (Hobbs, 1990).

The *usnic acid* in usnea is effective against gram-positive bacteria, such as streptococcus and staphylococcus, making usnea a valuable addition to herbal formulas for sore throats and skin infections. It is also effective against a bacterium that commonly causes pneumonia. Recent animal trials have demonstrated that usnic acid can reduce pain and lower fever (Okuyama et al., 1995).

Some conditions for which usnea has been used in European research are (Hobbs, 1990):

athlete's foot
bacterial infection
bronchitis
burns
colds
flu
fungus infection
lupus erythematosus

mastitis
pneumonia
ringworm
sinus infection
tuberculosis
urinary tract infection
vaginal infection (trichomonas)

Usnea should be taken as a tincture or a salve. I recommend combining it with herbs such as echinacea, yerba
mansa, or osha when treating colds, flu, and sore throats
when bacterial infection is suspected. It is indispensable in
the treatment of strep throat, and can eliminate the need for
antibiotics. If your sore throat lasts longer than about a
week, and you don't successfully treat it with herbs, be sure
to see a physician. Usnea can also be combined with uva ursi
when treating urinary tract infections.

Uva Ursi, Bearberry
(Arctostaphylos uva ursi)

Uva ursi is a classic urinary tract tonic and anti-
infective. The constituent *arbutin* in uva ursi breaks down in
the body to form the antibiotic constituent *hydroquinone*,
which is excreted through the urinary tract. The antibiotic
constituent thus has no undesired effect on the intestinal
bacteria, and is delivered directly to whatever bacteria are in
the bladder or urethra. Echinacea is, of course, an immune
system stimulant. Combining the herbs attacks the bacteria
directly via hydroquinone in the urine, while echinacea
strengthens the innate resistance.

BOX 19.1
CLINICAL PROPERTIES AND USES OF UVA URSI

(Source: Kirkbride, 1996)

PROPERTIES

Influences all the mucous membranes, but especially genitourinary tract

Astringent and tonic to the urinary tract

Tonification of the pelvic organs, male or female

USES

catarrh in the bladder
flaccid vagina and uterus
leukorrhea in females
prolapsed uterus
prostatic weakness
ulceration of the bladder and kidneys
urinary tract conditions

There is more to uva ursi than bacteria-killing ability. Canadian naturopath and chiropractor Douglas Kirkbride is a master herbalist, with more than forty years of clinical experience. In a 1991 lecture, he described one herb from each of the major therapeutic herb categories—the one herb that he simply couldn't do without. For urinary tract herbs, he chose uva ursi. Box 19.1 shows some of the conditions for which he has found uva ursi useful. Kirkbride suggests taking uva ursi as a tea in the following formula as a urinary tract tonic.

uva ursi	1 ounce
squaw vine	1 ounce
(*Mitchella repens*)	
dandelion root	1 ½ ounces
(*Taraxacum off.*)	

Simmer in one quart of water for twenty minutes. Strain and give four-tablespoon doses three times a day

It is best to avoid using uva ursi in cases of chronic kidney inflammation. I know of one confirmed case in which it caused elevations of creatinine in such a condition, verified by rechallenge—an indication of worsening the inflammation (Tilgner, 1996).

CASE STUDY: URINARY TRACT INFECTION A patient of mine was a thirty-eight-year-old woman complaining of a ten-month continuous urinary tract infection. A single species of fecal bacteria had been found in her urine upon lab testing by an M.D. The infection had been treated unsuccessfully with antibiotics for ten months. I suggested the following treatment:

FORMULA

uva ursi	1 ounce
echinacea angustifolia	1 ounce
nettle leaf (*Urtica dioica*)	30 drops

One dropperful three times a day.

Upon follow-up two months later, the patient said that the original infection had cleared in six days, and she remained asymptomatic for two months following. Mild symptoms began to return after two months, and lab tests showed that fecal bacteria had again begun to grow in the urinary tract.

I have described twenty-two herbs, including echinacea and goldenseal. The next chapter describes uses for them for common medical conditions.

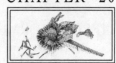

CHAPTER 20

HERBAL APPLICATIONS FOR SPECIFIC CONDITIONS

Before I describe some home treatments with herbs for various conditions, let me emphasize this: If you are sick with anything other than a short-term self-limiting illness, see a physician or other licensed health care practitioner. If you do not want to undergo the treatments of conventional medicine, at least get a proper diagnosis or consult a licensed practitioner of alternative medicine. See Appendix C for a list of these. Licensed naturopathic physicians, listed there, hold a doctoral degree from a four-year naturopathic medical college. They are the best-trained physicians in the country in a wide variety of alternative therapies, including medical herbalism. They also offer complete diagnostic and referral skills.

HERBAL FORMULAS AND "SIMPLES"

Most herbalists do not prescribe single herbs, but combine several herbs in a formula. Three or more herbs are mixed together, and their combined effects are more potent than any one of them would be alone for your condition. A skilled herbalist will devise a formula specifically for you—for your constitution, your condition, and the stage of your illness. On a return visit, the herbalist may modify the formula for your changing state.

Echinacea, goldenseal, and the other herbs discussed in this book often appear in commercial formulas in health food stores. Many of these are excellent, but they have several drawbacks. First, they are often not tailored to your specific condition. Second, they may contain only small amounts of the herb or herbs that you need the most. For instance, if a formula contains six herbs in equal parts, you are only getting five drops of each herb in a thirty-drop dose. To get the appropriate dose of one or two of the key herbs, you may need to take a teaspoonful of the formula. For commercial tinctures, typically costing eight to ten dollars an ounce, this becomes very expensive. You can reduce this cost by making your own tinctures and combining them (see Appendix A), or by purchasing several tinctures and making simple formulas.

Simples are herb formulas containing fewer herbs—two or three—and sometimes only a single herb. They are easy to prepare, and they ensure that you get an adequate dose of the key herbs in the simple. In this chapter, I'll describe some simples you can use, either as tinctures or as teas, for a wide variety of medical conditions.

Use one or more suggestions from the list offered. For more specific information on how to use the herbs in the formulas, consult the following chapters:

echinacea	Chapter 11
goldenseal	Chapter 14
barberry	Chapter 15
coptis	
Oregon grape root	
yerba mansa	
boneset	Chapter 17
black elder	
osha	
licorice	Chapter 18
reishi	
Siberian ginseng	
burdock	Chapter 19
cleavers	
red root	
usnea	
uva ursi	

ACNE

- Drink burdock root tea. Place an ounce of dried burdock root in a quart of water and simmer for twenty minutes. Drink the quart throughout the day.
- If the acne is infected, apply an echinacea wash. Dilute one part of echinacea tincture in three parts of water. Apply with a gauze pad every several hours.

AUTOIMMUNE DISORDERS

- Be sure to consult a medical practitioner for ongoing monitoring of the state of your illness.
- Make a tea of reishi mushroom and licorice root. Place an ounce of reishi and a half-ounce of licorice root in two quarts of water. Simmer for several hours or until the water is reduced by about one-third. Drink three cups a day for three weeks, then take a week or two off. Large amounts of licorice taken persistently can cause high blood pressure and salt imbalances in the body.
- Make a tea of the following digestive herbs, in equal parts: peppermint *(Mentha piperita)*, chamomile *(Chamomilla recutita)*, fennel seed *(Foeniculum vulgare)*, licorice root, and slippery elm *(Ulmus fulva)*. Place a handful of each in two quarts of water or in the bottom of an automatic drip coffee maker. Simmer for a half-hour. Drink two or three cups a day.
- Take a fluid extract of Siberian ginseng, four dropperfuls a day. See Chapter 18 for details.
- Make your own unsweetened fresh applesauce for daily consumption, or buy apple pectin at a health food store.
- Stop taking the above treatments during an acute outbreak or fever. Instead, take echinacea in doses of fifteen to twenty drops every two to three hours for up to a week. You may also take three or four cups of burdock tea a day (see recipe under Acne).

BITES AND STINGS

- Apply an echinacea wash at full tincture strength.
- Apply an echinacea-and-clay poultice. See Chapter 11 for a recipe.
- Also take echinacea internally, a dropperful every two hours.
- Take burdock root tea internally (see recipe under Acne).
- An alternative external application is a garlic wash or poultice. An ancient remedy for scorpion sting is to chew a clove of garlic, mix it well with saliva, and apply it to the wound. Don't leave garlic in place for more than twenty minutes, because it can cause skin burns.

BOILS AND CARBUNCLES

- Make a tea of equal parts of burdock root and stinging nettle *(Urtica dioica)*. Put a handful of each in a quart of water and simmer for twenty minutes. Strain and drink the quart throughout the day.
- Apply echinacea tincture diluted with an equal part of water. Apply on a gauze pad and tape in place. Renew the compress every few hours.
- Take echinacea internally, a dropperful every two or three hours.

BRONCHITIS

Dry, Inflamed, Acute Bronchitis

Mix equal parts of tinctures of echinacea, usnea, and licorice. Take two dropperfuls every three hours. Drink plenty of water.

Simple Bronchitis, with Productive Cough

- Mix equal parts of echinacea, Oregon grape, usnea, and osha. Take two dropperfuls in a cup of warm water every three hours.
- Make a tea of black elder flowers, boneset, and licorice root. Place a handful of each in a quart of water, and simmer, covered well, for ten minutes. Let tea cool to room temperature. Take a half-cup every three or four hours.
- Take garlic-honey syrup. Peel five or six garlic heads and pulverize them in a blender. Add enough warm honey (warm enough to make it runny) to cover, and blend again. Let it sit overnight. Take a tablespoon four times a day.

Bronchitis with Lymphatic Swelling and a Productive Cough

Mix equal parts of echinacea, usnea, and red root tinctures with a half-part of boneset. Take two dropperfuls every three hours for up to three days. If lymphatic swelling persists, see a physician.

Bronchitis with Discharge of Yellow or Green Phlegm

Mix echinacea tincture with an equal amount of tincture of goldenseal or Oregon grape root. Take a dropperful in some warm water every three hours.

Chronic Bronchitis

- Make a tea of reishi mushroom and licorice. See instructions under Autoimmune Disorders, above.
- Mix two parts of echinacea tincture with one part of boneset tincture. Take a dropperful every three or four hours. Don't take the boneset for more than about a week.

BURNS

Cool down a sunburn or second-degree burn (with blisters) with an echinacea wash: one part of tincture to six parts water. Dab on with a gauze pad. Renew every half-hour for four or five treatments, and then as needed to reduce the inflammation. Third-degree burns, with tissue damage, require prompt medical attention.

CANCERS

Despite years of searching, I have yet to find a reliable herbal treatment for cancer. A handful of herbally cured cases exist, but they are exceptions. The most successful treatments of advanced cancer include both conventional and alternative treatments. Herbal and other alternative treatments can reduce the side effects of conventional treatments such as radiation and chemotherapy.

- Make a soup of astragalus, reishi, burdock root, and licorice. Put one ounce each of the astragalus, reishi, and burdock with a half-ounce of licorice root in three quarts of water. Simmer for several hours, or until one-third of the water is gone. Take three cups a day.
- Take a simple tea of burdock root, red clover blossoms, and licorice. Place a handful each of the burdock and red clover with about half that amount of licorice in a quart of water. Simmer, covered tightly, for ten minutes, and let cool to room temperature. Take three to four cups a day.
- Include garlic in the diet as can be tolerated, up to three cloves a day, either raw or cooked. Take the garlic cocktail described in Chapter 16.
- Take ginger tea for nausea accompanying cancer or chemotherapy. Slice up a thumb-sized piece of fresh ginger root *(Zingiber officinalis)* in a quart of water. Simmer, covered, for twenty minutes. Sip as needed.
- Take echinacea for pain in advanced cancer, up to a half-ounce of the tincture a day.

COLDS OR FLU

See a detailed description in Table 17.1.

Diarrhea and Dysentery

- Do not suppress acute diarrhea with over-the-counter medications or with drying, astringent herbs. The diarrhea is washing out the infectious agents and their toxins, and suppressing it may make you sicker.

- For simple diarrhea, drink peppermint tea. Pour boiling water over a handful of peppermint leaves in a quart jar and screw the lid on tightly. Let it cool, overnight if convenient. Take up to four cups a day.

- For prevention while traveling in foreign countries, take fifteen drops of goldenseal, or any of its berberine-containing substitutes listed in Chapter 15, two or three times a day, provided bitter tonics are not contraindicated for your constitution (see Chapter 12 for contraindications).

- For food poisoning or "bad water" while traveling, with accompanying nausea, drink garlic-and-ginger tea. Simmer three cloves of garlic and an equal amount of fresh ginger in a quart of water. Drink the quart throughout the day, as tolerated; the garlic can be irritating.

- For dysentery, take fifteen drops of a goldenseal tincture or one of its berberine-containing substitutes every three or four hours.

- For chronic dysentery, take goldenseal tincture or a combination of Oregon grape root and yerba mansa: one dropperful four times a day.

- For dysentery from parasitic infections, consult a physician for a diagnosis. Some parasites, including the one responsible for amoebic dysentery, can have serious systemic complications, such as liver abscess. Consult a practitioner of natural medicine (see Appendix C) for advice on treating parasites.

EAR INFECTIONS

- Take a tincture of equal parts of echinacea and Oregon grape root, one dropperful every two or three hours. For an infant over eight months old, give three or four drops.
- Remove milk from the diet, and see if the "infection" goes away. Allergy to dairy products is a common cause of ear congestion in children.

ECZEMA

- Use black elder flower tea. Add two handfuls of the flowers to a quart jar. Fill the jar with boiling water and screw the lid on tightly. Let it cool to room temperature. Use as a wash for the eczema, and also take a half-cup internally three or four times a day. Continue for at least ten days.
- Use burdock and cleavers tea. Put a handful of each in a quart of boiling water. Simmer for ten minutes. Let cool to room temperature. Drink three or four cups a day. Burdock increases circulation to the skin, and in some instances this may irritate the eczema.
- Take a mixture of equal parts of echinacea and Oregon grape root tincture internally, a dropperful

every three hours. Also apply the tincture mixture, diluted in three parts of water, directly to the eczema.

- If the eczema is infected and oozing, apply goldenseal tincture, diluted in three parts of water, directly to the eczema.
- Use the digestive formula listed under Autoimmune Disorders above.
- Moisten some powder of slippery elm root and apply as a poultice for its soothing effect.

EYE INFECTIONS

- Make an eyewash of a dropperful of a strong tea of goldenseal in a pint of water.
- Make a similar eyewash of Oregon grape or coptis.
- Take echinacea internally, a dropperful every two or three hours.

FOOD POISONING

Take garlic-and-ginger tea (see recipe under Diarrhea).

GUM DISEASE WITH LOOSE TEETH

Mix equal parts of tinctures of echinacea, goldenseal, and myrrh *(Commiphora myrrha)*. Dilute a teaspoon in an ounce of water. Swirl around thoroughly in the mouth and hold until it has been absorbed by the tissues. Repeat four or five times a day.

HERPES

- At the first prodromal symptoms, take echinacea, in teaspoon doses, every two hours. This may abort the outbreak.
- If the herpes has already erupted, take osha tincture internally, in dropperful doses every three or four hours. Also apply the tincture directly to the sore.
- Blend three cloves of garlic in a tolerable medium such as orange or carrot juice, and take it as a single dose. Repeat the dose twice a day.
- Blend a clove or two of garlic in a cup of wine and let it sit overnight. Use it frequently as a wash.

INFECTED WOUNDS

- Take echinacea internally, a dropperful of tincture every two or three hours.
- Disinfect the wound with echinacea tincture, diluted in three parts of water, applied with a gauze pad. Keep an echinacea-soaked gauze pad in place on the wound with a bandage. Change every two hours.
- Same as above, but mix the echinacea with an equal part of Oregon grape root tincture.
- Blend a clove or two of garlic in a cup of wine and let it sit overnight. Use it frequently as a wash and compress, like the echinacea solution described above.

NASAL CATARRH
(CHRONIC RUNNY NOSE)

- Mix equal parts of tinctures of echinacea, usnea, and yerba mansa. Take a dropperful every three hours.
- Dilute a dropperful of goldenseal in six parts of water, and snort it into the nasal passages.
- Make a tea of equal parts of boneset and elderberry. Put a handful of each in a quart jar, fill with boiling water, and screw the lid on tightly. Let it cool to room temperature. Take a half cup four times a day.

PEMPHIGUS VULGARIS

Apply echinacea as with Infected Wounds above, or apply a clay poultice as described in Chapter 11.

POISON IVY AND POISON OAK

- Apply an echinacea wash, with the tincture diluted in three parts of water.
- Make a very thin clay application as described in Chapter 11. Add enough water that the mixture is thin enough to "paint" on the outbreak.

SKIN ULCERS

- Keep the area moist with echinacea tincture, diluted in three parts of water.

- Apply goldenseal, or any of its substitutes listed in Chapter 15, in the same way.

SORE THROAT AND STREP THROAT

- Mix equal parts of tinctures of echinacea, osha, and usnea in a little water. Put two dropperfuls in a little water. Every two or three hours, gargle for a while and then swallow.
- If the mucous membranes are infected and oozing, take goldenseal, or a combination of Oregon grape and yerba mansa tinctures in the same way, but with one dropperful in the water instead of two.

STAPH INFECTIONS

- Mix equal parts of echinacea and Oregon grape tinctures. Take a dropperful every two to three hours. Also apply directly to the infection with the same frequency. Apply with a gauze pad and tape it in place. Change the dressing frequently. A persistent or worsening infection requires medical attention.
- Apply usnea tincture directly to the infection in the same manner.
- Blend a clove or two of garlic in a cup of wine, and let sit overnight. Apply externally in the same manner.

TONSILLITIS

- Mix equal parts of tinctures of echinacea and usnea in some water, and apply as described under Sore Throat, above.
- Boil two tablespoons of red root in a quart of water for twenty minutes. Let it cool. Add two tablespoons of echinacea tincture. Then take one-third of the quart an hour before each meal, mixing or shaking well before drinking.
- With yellow or green mucous discharge, take a dropperful of goldenseal tincture in some warm water and gargle every three hours. You can substitute equal parts of Oregon grape and yerba mansa for the goldenseal, and apply two-dropper doses in the same manner.

URINARY TRACT INFECTIONS

- Be sure to consult a physician for persistent symptoms.
- Mix equal parts of the tinctures of echinacea and uva ursi. Take a dropperful every three hours. If symptoms persist past a week, consult a physician. Don't take uva ursi for longer than about ten days.
- With mucous discharge, take two dropperfuls of a tincture of equal parts of Oregon grape root, uva ursi, and yerba mansa four times a day in warm water.
- For pain and irritation, take one of the above along with a tea of marshmallow root or hollyhock flowers (*Althea officinalis, Althea rosea*).

VAGINAL INFECTIONS

- Make a douche of any of the following herbs (or combine them), adding one dropperful of tincture per cup of warm water: echinacea, usnea, goldenseal.
- Blend three peeled garlic cloves in three pints of water. Strain through cheesecloth. Apply as a douche.

MAKING YOUR OWN TINCTURES AND TEAS

You can save money and become more involved in your own self-care by purchasing whole herbs through a health food store, herb shop, or mail-order catalog. I list some sources for mail-order herbs in Appendix B.

TINCTURES

A tincture is a solution of herbal material in a mixture of alcohol and water. The herb is soaked in the solution for about three weeks, extracting many of the medicinal properties of the plant. Tinctures are so expensive at retail—eight to twelve dollars per ounce—that cost may be an issue if you want to take them on an ongoing basis or in higher doses. It is very easy to make your own tinctures; it takes about the same effort as preparing a meal, and you can save about three-fourths of the price of a commercial tincture. Here's all you need:

ALCOHOL   Purchase grain alcohol from a liquor store. The kind I am most familiar with is 190-proof, or ninety-five percent alcohol. Grain alcohol may be illegal in your state. If this is the case, you can use a commercial liquor such as vodka. It should be at least eighty proof, or forty percent alcohol.

HERBAL MATERIAL   Purchase the herb in as whole a form as possible, such as the whole roots or leaves, rather than as powders.

Preparation

1. Dilute the alcohol to make an alcohol-water mixture with approximately sixty percent alcohol (it does not have to be precise). For 190-proof grain alcohol, put two-and-a-half cups of the alcohol in a quart jar and fill it with water.
2. Break up the herbs by cutting, chopping, blending, or grinding them as small as possible. However, they should not be a fine powder.
3. Place the herbs in a jar with a tight-fitting lid, and cover with the alcohol. Fasten the lid and keep in a cool dark place.
4. Every day, take the bottle out and turn or shake it to be sure the herbs and the solvent are well mixed. Sometimes the herbs will absorb the solvent, leaving more room at the top of the bottle. You can add more solvent if this occurs.

5. After about three weeks, empty the contents and strain the solvent from the herbal material. You can squeeze out every last drop using a tincture press. A variety of sizes of press are available from the companies listed in Appendix B, including an inexpensive cloth-and-dowel press from Longevity Herbs in White Salmon, Washington.

Teas

Teas are of two kinds: infusions and decoctions.

Infusions

Infusions are made of the more fragile plant parts, such as leaves and flowers. The secret to making a good infusion is to dissolve as much of the plant constituents as you can in hot water, but not destroy those constituents or drive away volatile ones by using too much heat. When you make a cup of peppermint tea, and you smell the nice aroma wafting through the room, you are smelling the escaping medicinal constituents.

The best way to make a strong infusion is to put an ounce or two of the herb in a quart canning jar. Pour in boiling water to fill the jar and fasten the cover tightly. This will prevent the volatile constituents from escaping. Let it cool to room temperature, from three to six hours. This long soaking will extract a maximum amount of the constituents. For convenience, prepare the tea at night before bedtime, and it will be cooled and ready in the morning. Strain and store what you don't drink right away in the refrigerator.

Decoctions

Decoctions are made from the harder parts of the plant, such as roots or seeds. Decoctions require longer cooking than infusions. Again, put an ounce or two of the plant part in a quart or two of water. Avoid using an iron pot. Bring just to a boil, and then keep on the lowest heat for twenty minutes, with a lid on the pot. Again, let the decoction cool to room temperature to extract the maximum amount of the constituents. Strain and store what you don't drink in the refrigerator.

MODERN TOOLS

It has never been easier to make batches of teas than at the present, due to the number of cooking implements and tools available to us. Here are some tips:

- First thing in the morning, make your infusion for the day in a French press coffee maker (available in any good coffee store), pouring boiling water over the herbs. Take your morning shower or make your other preparations for the day. Then, before going out the door, strain and pour the infusion into a thermos bottle. You will then have warm tea throughout the day.
- Make your decoctions in an automatic-drip coffee maker with a hot plate. Place the herbs in the *bottom* of the coffee maker, not where the coffee would usually go. Then add water to the top of the machine, and let the preheated water run over the herbs. Let the decoction sit on the warmer for twenty to thirty minutes. Strain and put in a thermos to take to work, or store in the refrigerator.

SOURCES OF HERBS, SEEDS, AND SUPPLIES

Many companies in North America make excellent herbal products, and I cannot name them all here. These are the sources I am personally most familiar with. If a company you like is not listed here, please don't assume that it is because I think they have poor-quality or unreliable products. Among the sources listed here, be sure to comparison-shop. Some have much better prices than others.

Frontier Herb Cooperative
P.O. Box 299
Norway, IA 52318
800-717-4372

Frontier is primarily a distributor of Western bulk herbs, spices, tinctures, and herb products and supplies. They also sell Asian and American ginseng in several grades, and all of the tonic herbs discussed in Chapter 18. This is the best full-service mail-order company.

Dancing Willow Herbs
960 Main Avenue
Durango, CO 81301
970-247-1654

Dancing Willow makes a line of high-quality tinctures, including the polysaccharide-enhanced echinacea tincture described in Chapter 11.

GAIA Herbs
62 Old Littleton Road
Harvard, MA 01451
800-831-7780

Gaia specializes in high-quality tinctures, fluid extracts, and concentrated herb preparations.

HerbPharm
P.O. Box 116
Williams, OR 97544
800-348-4372

HerbPharm makes high-quality tinctures, fluid extracts, and concentrated preparations. Their Siberian ginseng product is the only one I am aware of made to the specifications of the Russian Pharmacopoeia. Most other commercial preparations are much weaker than those used in Russia, where the tonic properties of the herb were perfected, and they won't yield their adaptogenic effects unless you take them in very high doses. HerbPharm concentrates the Russian formulation to double-strength.

Turtle Island Herbs
412 Boulder Street
Boulder, CO 80302
303-442-2215

Turtle Island sells a full line of high-quality tinctures and formulas.

Wise Woman Herbals
P.O. Box 279
Creswell, OR 97426
800-532-5219

Wise Woman Herbals sells a full line of high-quality tinctures and has an extensive line of prepared formulas.

Ginseng Roots, Bulk Chinese Herbs, and Asian Immune-Tonic Formulas

East Earth Tradewinds
P.O. Box 493151
Redding, CA 96049-3151
800-258-6878
Fax: 800-258-1384

White Crane
426 First Street
Jersey City, NJ 07302
800-994-3721
Internet: crane@inch.com

East Earth Herb, Inc.
P.O. Box 2802
Eugene, OR 97402
800-827-4372
Fax: 503-485-7347

Seeds

Abundant Life Seed Foundation
P.O. Box 772
Port Townsend, WA 98368
360-385-5660

Otto Richter and Sons
Goodwood
Ontario L0C 1A0
Canada
905-666-3697

See also the catalog from Frontier Herb listed above.

Tincture Presses

Life Force Herbal Press
P.O. Box 4987
Boulder, CO 80306
303-642-0960

Longevity Herb Company
1549 Jewett
White Salmon, WA 98672

Books

American Botanical Council
P.O. Box 201660
Austin, TX 78720-1660
512-331-8868

Eclectic Medical Publications
2125 NW Division
Gresham, OR 97030
800-332-4372

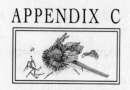

WHERE TO FIND A PRACTITIONER OF NATURAL MEDICINE

To find a physician who practices natural and herbal medicine, try the following referral resources.

American Association of Acupuncture and Oriental Medicine
433 Front Street
Catasauqua, PA 18032
610-433-2448

American Association of Naturopathic Physicians
2366 Eastlake Avenue East, Suite 322
Seattle, WA 98102
206-323-7610

American College of Advancement in Medicine
P.O. Box 3427
Laguna Hills, CA 92654
714-583-7666

Canadian Association of Ayurvedic Medicine
P.O. Box 749, Station B
Ottawa, Ontario K1P 5P8
Canada

Herb Research Foundation
1007 Pearl Street, Suite 200
Boulder, CO 80302
800-748-2617

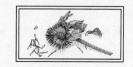

GLOSSARY

IMMUNE SYSTEM TERMS

See Chapter 4 for a more detailed description of the immune system.

Antibodies Small proteins that circulate throughout the blood, extracellular fluid, and lymph, which are designed to attach to, neutralize, or destroy specific antigens. They are produced by B-cells or plasma cells.

Antigens Foreign particles that elicit an immune response from B-cells or T-cells. The cells are pre-programmed to attack one specific antigen.

B-lymphocytes (B-cells) Cells of the specific immune system which identify particular antigens and produce antibodies. The B-cells are transformed, with the assistance of the T-helper cells, into plasma cells, which produce huge amounts of antibodies.

Cell-Mediated Immunity Immunity involving the T-cells. Healthy cell-mediated immunity is necessary for the optimal functioning of humoral immunity.

Complement A set of chemicals that circulates freely in the blood and the extracellular fluid. It may trigger other parts of the immune system, including an inflammatory response or may destroy invaders directly.

Cytotoxic T-cells See Natural Killer Cells.

Fever Response A beneficial response triggered by secretions of the phagocytes. Fever promotes the rapid multiplication of immune system cells and enhances tissue repair.

Humoral-Mediated Immunity Immunity involving the B-cells and antibodies to specific antigens. Humoral immunity requires the participation of the T-4 helper cells to function efficiently.

Hyaluronic Acid/Hyaluronidase Hyaluronic acid is secreted into the extracellular fluid matrix and tends to thicken it into a gel. This provides a barrier to invading organisms. Hyaluronidase thins the gel. The balance between the two determines the thickness of the gel.

Immunity The body's ability to repel invading organisms and dispose of its own wastes while maintaining the integrity of biological "self."

Inflammation A response of the immune system that prevents the spread of invading organisms, removes pathogens and dead cells, attracts phagocytes and members of the specific immune defense to the area, and promotes tissue repair. The classic characteristics of inflammation are swelling, pain, heat, and redness. Chronic inflammation may cause scarring and profound tissue changes.

Macrophages   Literally "big eaters"—large phagocytes that have the capacity to engulf many invading organisms. They reside in or are attached to the tissues.

Monocytes   Phagocytes that circulate in the blood. They migrate to the scene of an infection in response to chemical triggers in the local area. Some monocytes enter the tissues and may become macrophages.

Natural Killer Cells   T-cells that attack virally infected cells, cancerous cells, and foreign cells such as are found in organ transplants. Technically, the T-cells are part of the specific cell-mediated immune system, but they may also act in a non-specific way against some invaders or cells.

Neutrophils   Phagocytes that circulate in the blood and migrate to the scene of an infection in response to a chemical trigger in the local area.

Phagocytes   Cells that surround and engulf invading organisms or extracellular debris. Phagocytes may also, after ingesting the organism, trigger other parts of the immune system.

Plasma cells   B-cells that have been transformed into antibody-producing factories, collectively producing billions of circulating antibodies to the antigen that initially triggered the B-cell. B-cells require the participation of T-helper cells to accomplish this transformation.

Specific Immune System A system including the B-cells, T-cells, and antibodies. Cells or antibodies are produced to kill invaders or cells containing specific proteins or other materials on their coats.

T-Helper Cells These respond only to antigens "handed" to them by phagocytes. The helper cell then emits chemicals that cause the proliferation of other T-helper cells, plasma cells, and antibodies. They attract still more phagocytes, drive them into a "feeding frenzy," and stimulate T-killer cells in the area. T-helper cell levels decline in AIDS patients, leaving them vulnerable to cancers and opportunistic infections.

T-Killer Cells See Natural Killer Cells.

White Blood Cells The cells in the blood, lymph, and extracellular fluid that are specialized elements of the immune system.

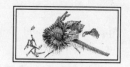

REFERENCES

Abudllah, T., Kirkpatrick, D.V., Williams, L., Carter, J. "Garlic as an intimicrobial and immune modulator in AIDS." Int Conf AIDS. 1989 Jun 4–9;5:466 (abstract no. Th.B.P.304).

Abdullah, T. "Garlic." *Prevention*, August 1987. Cited In: Heinerman, J. *The Healing Benefits of Garlic: From Pharaohs to Pharmacists*. New Canaan, Connecticut: Keat Publishing. 1994.

Adetumbi, M.A., Lau, D.H. "*Allium sativum* (garlic) a natural antibiotic." *Med Hypotheses* 1983 Nov;12(3):227–37.

Adetumbi, M., Javor, G.T., Lau, B.H. "*Allium sativum* (garlic) inhibits lipid synthesis by Candida albicans." *Antimicrob Agents Chemother* 1986 Sep;30(3): 499–501.

AIDS Research Alliance. "Garlic for cryptosporidiosis?" *Treat Rev* 1996 Aug;(No 22):11.

Akhter, M.H., Sabir, M., and Bhide, N.K. "Anti–inflammatory effect of berberine in rats injected locally with cholera toxin." *Indian J Med Res* 1977 Jan;65(1):133–41.

Amin, A.H., Subbaiah, T.V., and Abbasi K.M. "Berberine sulfate: antimicrobial activity, bioassay, and mode of action." *Can J Microbiol* 1969; 15:1067–1076.

Amman, M. and Suter, K. *Deutsch Apoth Zeit* 1987;127:853.

Anesini, C. and Perez, C. "Screening of plants used in Argentine folk medicine for antimicrobial activity." *J Ethnopharmacol* 1993 Jun;39(2):119–28.

Anonymous. "Fail to snooze, immune cells lose." *Sci News* 1995;147:11.

Appleton, J.A. and Tansey, M.R. "Inhibition of growth of zoopathogenic fungi by garlic extract." *Mycologia* 1975 Jul–Aug;67(4):882–5.

Awang, D.V.C. and Kindack, D.G. "Echinacea." *Can Pharm J.* 1991;124: 512–516.

Babbar, O.P., Chatwal, V.K., Ray, I.B., Mehra, M.K. "Effect of berberine chloride eye drops on clinically positive trachoma patients." *Indian J Med Res* 1982;76(Suppl):83–88.

Baenkler, H.W. "Exercise and the immune system: the impact on diseases." *Rheumatic Diseases Sport Rheumatology.* 1992;15:5–21.

Baker, R.C., and Jerrells, T.R. "Recent developments in alcoholism: immunological aspects." *Recent Dev Alcohol* 1993;11:249–71.

Barton, Benjamin Smith. *"Collections for an Essay Towards a Materia Medica of the United States."* Bulletin of the Lloyd Library, No.1 Reproduction Series, No.1. 1798 and 1804 (reprint two volumes in one) Cincinnati, Ohio: Lloyd Library, 1900.

Bauer, R., Khan, I., Lotter, H., Wagner, H. "Structure and Stereochemistry of new sesquiterpene esters from *Echinacea purpurea* (L.) Moench." *Helv. Chim. Acta* 1985;68:2355–2358.

Bauer, R., Khan, I., Wagner, H. "Echinacea drugs. Standardization with HPLC and TLC." *Deutsch Apoth Ztng* 1986;126:1065–1070. [Cited in Awang et al.]

Bauer, R., Khan, I., Jurcic, K., Wagner, H. "Immunologically active sesquiterpene esters from *Parthenium integrifolium* an adulterant of *Echinacea purpurea*." Poster presented at Biologically Active Natural Products Symposium, Phytochemical Society of Europe, Lausanne, Switzerland, 3–5 Sept, 1986.

Bauer, R. and Wagner, H. "Comments on the echinacea problem." *Amer Herb Assoc Quart Newsletter* 1987;5(4):4.

Bauer, R., Khan, I.A., Wagner, H. "TLC and HPLC analysis of *Echinacea pallida* and *Echinacea angustifolia* roots." *Planta Medica* 1988;54:426–430.

Bauer, R., Jurcic, K., Puhlmann, J., Wagner, H. "Immunologische in vivo- und in vitro-Untersuchungen mit *Echinacea*-Extrakten." *Arzneimittel Forschung* 1988;38(1):276–281.

Bauer, R., Remiger, P., Jurcic, K., Wagner, H. "Beinflussung der Phagozytoseaktivität durch *Echinacea*-Extrakte." *Zeitschrift für Phytotherapie* 1989; 10:43–48.

Bauer, R. and Wagner, H. *Echinacea: Handbuch für Ärzte, Apotheker, und andere Naturwissenschaftler.* Stuttgart: Wissenschaftliche Verlagsgessellschaft, mbH, 1990.

Bauer, R. and Wagner, H. "*Echinacea* species as potential immunostimulatory drugs." In: *Economic and Medicinal Plant Research* v.5, Wagner, H. and Farnsworth, N.R., eds. New York: Academic Press, 1991.

Bauer, R. *Zeitschrift für Phytotherapie* 1996;17:251–252. Cited in: Bone, K. Phytomedicine Conference Report—Part 2. *MediHerb Monitor,* 1996;(November):1.

Beck, J.J. and Stermitz, F.R. *J. Natural Products* 1995;58(7):1047–1055.

Bensky, D. and Gamble, H. *Chinese Herbal Medicine: Materia Medica.* Seattle, Washington: Eastland Press, 1986.

Bergner, P. "The Best New Herbs." *East West.* August, 1986.

Bergner, P. "Contraindications for Echinacea?" *Medical Herbalism* 1990;2(3):6.

Bergner, P. "Top Herbs in Medical Practice." *Medical Herbalism* 1994;6(1):10.

Bergner, P. *The Healing Power of Ginseng and the Tonic Herbs.* Rocklin, CA: Prima Publishing, 1996.

Bernstein, J. Alpert, S. Nauss, K. and Suskind, R. "Depression of lymphocyte transformation following glucose ingestion." *Am J Clin Nutr* 1977;30:613.

Beuscher, N., Bodinet, C., Willigmann, I., and Egert, D. "Immunomodulierende Eigenschaften von Wurzelextrakten verschiedener *Echinacea*-Arten." *Zeitschrift für Phytotherapie* 1995;16;157–166.

Bhide, M.B., Chavan, S.R., Dutta, N.K. "Absorption, distribution and extretion of berberine." *Indian J Med Res* 1969;57:2128–2131.

Boericke, W. *Pocket Manual of Homeopathic Materia Medica.* New Delhi: Jain Publishers, 1922. Reprint edition,1984.

Bone, K. "Long-Term Use of Echinacea." *Medical Herbalism* 1995;7(1–2):23 [letter].

Borukh, I.F., Kirbaba, V.I., Demkevich, L.I., Barabash. O.Y. "Bactericidal action of volatile phytoncides of garlic." *Vopr Pitan* 1974 Sep–Oct;0(5):80–1.

Borukh, I.F., Kirbaba, V.I., Demkevich, L.I., Barabash, O.Y. "Bactericidal properties of volatile fractions of garlic phytoncids." *Prikl Biokhim Mikrobiol* 1975 May–Jun;11(3):478–9.

Boyle, W. *Herb Doctors: Pioneers in Nineteenth-Century American Botanical Medicine.* East Palestine, Ohio: Buckeye Naturopathic Press, 1988.

Boyle, W. *Official Herbs: Botanical Substances in the United States Pharmacopoeias 1820–1990J.* East Palestine, Ohio: Buckeye Naturopathic Press, 1991.

Bräunig, B., Dorn, M., Limburg, Knick, E., Bausendorf. "*Echinacea purpurea* radix for strengthening the immune response in flu-like infections." *Zeitschrift für Phytotherapie* 1992; 13:7–13.

Brody, J.A., Overfield, T., and Hammes, L.M. "Depression of the tuberculin reaction by viral vaccines." *NEJM* 1964;271:1294–1296.

Brosche, T., Platt, D., and Dorner, H. "The effect of a garlic preparation on the composition of plasma lipoproteins and erythrocyte membranes in geriatric subjects." *Br J Clin Pract* 1990;44:12–19.

Brosche, B. and Platt, D. "Garlic." *Br Med J* 1991;303:785.

Brosche, T., and Platt, N. "Knoblauchtherapie und zellulaere Immunabwehr im Alter." *Z. Phytother* 1994;15:23–24.

Byrd, R.C. "Positive therapeutic effects of intercessory prayer in a coronary care unit population." *South Med J* 1988;81(7):826–9.

Caporaso, N., Smith, S.M., Eng, R.H. "Antifungal activity in human urine and serum after ingestion of garlic *(Allium sativum)*." *Antimicrob Agents Chemother* 1983 May;23(5):700–2.

Carson, V.B. "Prayer, meditation, exercise, and special diets: behaviors of the hardy person with HIV/AIDS." *J Assoc Nurses AIDS Care* 1993;4(3):18–28.

Chan, E. "Displacement of bilirubin from albumin by berberine." *Biol Neonate* 1993;63(4):201–8.

Chen, H.C., Chang, M.D., Chang, T.J. "Antibacterial properties of some spice plants before and after heat treatment." *Chung Hua Min Kuo Wei Sheng Wu Chi Mien I Hsueh Tsa Chih* 1985 Aug;18(3):190–5.

Chopra, R.N., Dikshit, B.B., Chowhan, J.S. "Pharmacological action of berberine." *Ind J Med Res* 1932;19:1193–1203.

Choudry, V.P., Sabir, M., and Bhide, V.N. "Berberine in giardiasis." *Ind Pediatr* 1972; 9:143–146.

Chowdhury, A.K., Ahsan, M., Islam, S.N., Ahmed, Z.U. "Efficacy of aqueous extract of garlic and allicin in experimental shigellosis in rabbits." *Indian J Med Res* 1991 Jan;93:33–6.

Christopher, J.R. *School of Natural Healing*. Springville, Utah: Christopher Publications, 1976.

Clapp, A. "A report on medical botany . . ." *Transactions of the American Medical Association* 1852 5:698–906.

Clarke, J.H. *Practical Dictionary of Homeopathic Materia Medica*. London: 1902. Reprint, Bradford, Devon: Health Science Press, 1963.

Comings, I.M. *New Engl Bot Med Surg J* 1847;1:41. Cited in: Hobbs, C. *Echinacea: The Immune Herb*. Santa Cruz, California: Botanica Press, 1990.

Conner, D.E., Beuchat, L.R. "Sensitivity of heat–stressed yeasts to essential oils of plants." *Appl Environ Microbiol* 1984 Feb;47(2):229–33.

Cook, W. *The Physio-Medical Dispensatory: A Treatise on Therapeutics, Materia Medica, and Pharmacy in Accordance With the Principles of Physiological Medication*. Cincinnati, OH: Wm. H. Cook, 1869.

Cook, W. *The New Materia Medica*. Cincinnati, Ohio: Wm. H. Cook, 1892.

Couegniet, E.G. and Flek, F. "Immunomodulation with *Viscum album* and *Echiancea purpurea* extracts." *Onkologie* 1987;10(3):27–33.

Couegniet, E.G. and Kühnast. *Therapiewoche* 1986;36(33):3352–3358.

Crellin, J.K. and Philpott, J. *Herbal Medicine Past and Present, Volume II: A Reference Guide to Medicinal Plants*. Durham, North Carolina: Duke University Press, 1990.

Culbreth, D.C. *A Manual of Materia Medica and Pharmacology*. Philadelphia, Pennsylvania: Lea and Febiger, 1927.

D'Adamo, P. "Larch arabinogalactan." *J Naturopathic Med*. 1996;6(1):33–37.

Dale, D.C. and Federman, D.D. *Scientific American Medicine* 1995;7:Inf Dis:X 2–3.

Dankert, J., Tromp, T.F., de Vries, H., Klasen, H.J. "Antimicrobial activity of crude juices of *Allium ascalonicum, Allium cepa* and *Allium sativum*." *Zentralbl Bakteriol [Orig A]* 1979 Oct;245(1–2):229–39.

Daucus, S. "Boneset." *Medical Herbalism* 1995;7(4):10.

Davis, L.E., Shen, J.K., and Cai, Y. "Antifungal activity in human cerebrospinal fluid and plasma after intravenous administration of *Allium sativum*." *Antimicrob Agents Chemother* 1990;34(4):651–653.

Davis, T. "The research evidence on the power of prayer and healing." *Can J Cardiovasc Nurs* 1994;5(2):34–6.

Department of National Health and Welfare. Food and Drug Regulations — amendment (Schedule Number 705). *Canada Gazette* 1989;March 11: 1350–1359.

Deshpande, R.G., Khan, M.B., Bhat, D.A., Navalkar, R.G. "Inhibition of *Mycobacterium avium* complex isolates from AIDS patients by garlic *(Allium sativum)."* *J Antimicrob Chemother.* 1993 Oct;32(4):623–6.

Dharmananda, Subhuti. Personal communication. April, 1995.

Didry, N., Pinkas, M., Dubreuil, L. "Antibacterial activity of species of the genus Allium." *Pharmazie* 1987 Oct;42(10):687–8.

Duke, J.A. *Handbook of Medicinal Herbs.* Boca Raton, FL: CRC Press, 1985.

Eibl, M., Mannhalter, J.W., and Zlabinger, G. "Abnormal T-lymphocyte subpopulations in healthy subjects after tetanus booster immunization." *NEJM* 1984; 310:198–199 [letter].

Eichner, E.R. "Infection, immunity, and exercise: What to tell patients." *Physician Sports Med* 1993;21:125–133.

Ellingwood, Finley. *American Materia Medica, Therapeutics, and Pharmacognosy.* Chicago, Illinois, 1919. Reprinted in 1983 by Eclectic Medical Publications, Portland, Oregon.

Elsasser-Beile, U., Willenbacher, W., Bartsch, H.H., Gallati, H., et al. "Cytokine production in leukocyte cultures during therapy with Echinacea extract." *J Clin Lab Anal* 1996;10(6):441–5.

Engs, R.C., Aldo-Benson, M. "The association of alcohol consumption with self–reported illness in university students." *Psychol Rep* 1995 Jun;76(3 Pt 1):727–36.

Erichsen-Brown, C. *Medicinal and Other Uses of North American Plants: a historical survey with special reference to the Eastern Indian tribes.* New York: Dover Publications, 1979.

Facino, R.M., Carini, M., Aldini, G., Marinello, C., et al. "Direct characterization of caffeoyl esters with antihyaluronidase activity in crude extracts from *Echinacea angustifolia* roots by fast atom bombardment tandem mass spectrometry." *Farmaco* 1993; 48(10): 1447–61.

Facino, R.M., Carini, M., Aldini, G., Saibene L, et al. "Echinacoside and caffeoyl conjugates protect collagen from free radical-induced degradation: a potential use of Echinacea extracts in the prevention of skin photodamage." *Planta Med* 1995;61(6):510–4.

Farnsworth, N.R., Bingel, A.S., Cordell, G.A. et al. "Potential value of plants as sources of new antifertility agents." *Int J Pharm Sci* 1975;64:535–598.

Felter, H.W. and Lloyd, J.U. *King's American Dispensatory.* Cincinnati, Ohio, 1898. Reprinted 1983. Portland, Oregon: Eclectic Medical Publications.

Felter, H.W. *The Eclectic Materia Medica, Pharmacology, and Therapeutics.* Cincinnati, Ohio, 1922. Reprinted 1985. Portland, Oregon: Eclectic Medical Publications.

Feng, Z.H., Zhang, G.M., Hao, T.L., Zhou, B., Zhang, H., Jiang, Z.Y. "Effect of diallyl trisulfide on the activation of T-cell and macrophage-mediated cytotoxicity." *J Tongji Med Univ* 1994;14(3):142–7.

Fletcher, R.D., Parker, B., Hassett, M. "Inhibition of coagulase activity and growth of *Staphylococcus aureus* by garlic extracts." *Folia Microbiol (Praha)* 1974;19(6):494–7.

Fliermans, C.B. "Inhibition of Histoplasma capsulatum by garlic." *Mycopathol Mycol Appl* 1973 Jul 31;50(3):227–31.

Foster, S. "Herb traders beware." *Herbalgram* 1985(a);2(1):3.

Foster, S. "Echinacea—an honest appraisal." *Business of Herbs* 1985(b); (March/April):8–10.

Foster, S. "Echinacea quality control monograph—a literature review." American Herbal Products Association Standards Committee, 1987.

Foster, S. *Herbalgram* 1989;21;7,35.

Foster, S. *Echinacea: Nature's Immune Enhancer.* Rochester, Vermont: Healing Arts Press, 1991.

Fromtling, R.A. and Bulmer, G.S. "In vitro effect of aqueous extract of garlic *(Allium sativum)* on the growth and viability of *Cryptococcus neoformans.*" *Mycologia* 1978 Mar–Apr;70(2):397–405.

Gaertner, W. *Landarzt* 1968;39(3):125–134

Gaisbauer, M. and Zimmerman, W. *Natura Med* 1986;1:6–10.

Ghannoum, M.A. "Inhibition of Candida adhesion to buccal epithelial cells by an aqueous extract of *Allium sativum* (garlic)." *J Appl Bacteriol* 1990 Feb; 68(2):163–9.

Ghosh, A.K. "Effect of berberine chloride on *Leishmania donovani.*" *Ind J Med Res* 1983;78:407–416.

Gilani, A.H. and Janbaz, K.H. "Prevention of acetaminophen-induced liver damage by *Berberis aristata* leaves." *Biochem Soc Trans* 1992;20(4):347.

Gilmore, M.R. "A study of the ethnobotany of the Omaha Indians." *Collections Neb St His Soc* 1913;17:314–357.

Gonzalez-Fandos, E., Garcia-Lopez, M.L., Sierra, M.L., Otero, A. "Staphylococcal growth and enterotoxins (A–D) and thermonuclease synthesis in the presence of dehydrated garlic." *J Appl Bacteriol* 1994 Nov;77(5):549–52.

Gowen, S.L., Erskine, D., McAskill, R., Hawkins, D. "An assessment of the usage of non-prescribed medication by HIV." *Int Conf AIDS*. 1993 Jun 6–11;9(1):497 (abstract no. PO-B29-2174).

Graham, N.M.H. "Adverse effects of aspirin, acetominophen and ibuprofen on the immune function, viral shedding and clinical status in rhinovirus-infected volunteers." *J Inf Dis*; 1990;162:1277–1282.

Gray A. *A Manual of Botany of the Northeastern United States*. Boston: James Munroe and Company, 1848.

Grieve, M. *A Modern Herbal*. New York: Dover Publications, 1931.

Gronovius, L.T. *Flora Virginica*. 2nd ed. 1762. Reprint ed., Cambridge, Mass: Arnold Arboretum, 1946. [Cited in Foster, 1991.]

Gupta, S. "Use of berberine in the treatment of giardiasis." *Am J Dis Child* 1975;129:866.

Hale, E.M. *Materia Medica and Special Therapeutics of the New Remedies*. Fourth Edition. Chicago, Illinois: 1875. Reprinted by Jain Publishers, New Delhi, 1995.

Hansen, F. *Die Zeit* Number 20, May 10, 1996. Cited in: Bone, K. "Phytomedicine Conference Report — Part 2." *MediHerb Monitor* 1996;(November):1.

Hayden, F.V. "Botany." In *Report of the Secretary of War*. 35th Congress, 2nd Session, 1858-1879, Senate Executive Document, Vol. 3, No. 1, Part 3, pp. 726–747. Cited in Foster, S. *Echinacea: Nature's Immune Enhancer*. Rochester, Vermont: Healing Arts Press, 1991.

Heesen, W. and Schroeder, C. "Die Bedeutung des Echiancin in der Tuberculöse-Therapie." *Med Monatsschr* 1960;14:251–256.

Heesen, W. "Unspecifische Behandlungsmöglichkeiten bei tuberkulöse Erkrankungen." *Erfahrungsheilkunde* 1964;13(5):209–217. [Cited in Bauer and Wagner, 1990.]

Hering, Constantine. *The Guiding Symptoms of our Materia Medica* (ten volumes). Philadelphia, 1893. Reprint edition: New Delhi: Jain Publishers, 1995.

Hobbs, C. *The Echinacea Handbook*. Portland, OR: Eclectic Institute 1989.

Hobbs, C. *Echinacea: The Immune Herb*. Santa Cruz, California: Botanica Press, 1990.

Hobbs, C. *Usnea: The Herbal Antibiotic*. Santa Cruz, California: Botanica Press, 1990.

Johnson, C.C., Johnson, G., et al. "Toxicity of alkaloids to certain bacteria." *Acta Pharm Tox.* 1952;8:71–78.

Johnson, M.G. and Vaughn, R.H. "Death of *Salmonella typhimurium* and *Escherichia coli* in the presence of freshly reconstituted dehydrated garlic and onion." *Appl Microbiol* 1969 Jun;17(6):903–5.

Jones, E. *Definite Medication: Containing Therapeutic Facts Gleaned From Forty Years of Practice*. Boston, Massachusetts: Therapeutic Publishing Company, 1911a.

Jones, E. *Cancer: Its Causes, Symptoms, and Treatment*. Boston, Massachusetts: Therapeutic Publishing Company, 1911b.

Jurcic, K., Melchart, D., Holsmann, M., Martin, P., et al. "Zwei probandenstudien zur stimulierung der granulozytenphagozytose durch *echinacea*-extract-haltige präparate." *Zeitschrift für Phytotherapie* 1989;10:67–70.

Kabelik, J. "Antimicrobial properties of garlic." *Pharmazie* 1970 Apr;25(4): 266–70.

Kamsat, S.A. "Clinical trial with berberine hydrochloride for the control of diarrhoea in acute gastroenteritis." *J Assoc Phys India* 1967;15:525–529.

Kandil, O.M., Abdulla, T.H., and Elkadi, A. "Garlic and the immune system in humans: its effect on natural killer cells." *Fed Proc* 1987;46:441.

Kandil, O., Abdullah, T., Tabuni, A.M., and Elkadi, A. "Potential role of *Allium sativum* in natural cytotoxicity." *Arch AIDS Res* 1988;1:230–231.

Kassler, W.J., Blanc, P., Greenblatt, R. "The use of medicinal herbs by human immunodeficiency virus-infected patients." *Arch Intern Med.* 1991 Nov; 151(11):2281–8.

Khin-Maung, U., Myo-Khin, Nyunt-Nyunt-Wai, et al. "Clinical trial of berberine in acute watery diarrhoea." *Br Med J* 1985;2986;291:1601–1605.

King, J. and Newton, R.S. *The Eclectic Dispensatory of the United States of America.* Cincinnati, OH: H.W. Derby, 1852.

Kirkbride, D. Wisdom of an Elder. *Medical Herbalism* 1996;8(3):14–16.

Koch, Fr.E. *Arzn Forsch* 1952;2:464. [Cited in Bauer and Wagner, 1991.]

Koch, Fr.F. *Arzn Forsch* 1963;3:16. [Cited in Bauer and Wagner, 1991.]

Kortung, G.W. and Born, W. *Arzneimittel Forschung* 1954;4:424–426.

Kortung, G.W. and Rasp, K. *Medizinische* 1954;45:1504–1508.

Kumar, A., Sharma, V.D. "Inhibitory effect of garlic *(Allium sativum Linn.)* on enterotoxigenic *Escherichia coli.*" *Indian J Med Res* 1982 Dec;76 Suppl:66–70.

Kumazawa, Y., Itagaki, A., Fukumoto, M., et al. "Activation of peritoneal macrophages by berberine alkaloids in terms of induction of cytostatic activity." *Int J Immunopharmacol* 1984;6:587–592.

Kuts-Chereaux, A.W. *Naturae Medicina and Naturopathic Dispensatory.* Des Moines, Iowa: American Naturopathic Physicians and Surgeons Associations, 1953.

Lampe, K.F. "Berberine." In: De Smet, P.A.G.M., Keller, K., Hänsel, R. et al. *Adverse Effects of Herbal Drugs 1.* New York: Springer-Verlag, 1992.

Larrey, D. and Pageaux, G.P. "Herbs and mushrooms that are toxic to the liver." *Seminars in Liver Disease* 1995;15(3)183–188.

Lenk, W. *Zeitschrift für Phytotherapie* 1989;10:49–51.

Lewis, W.H. and Elvin-Lewis, M.P.F. *Medical Botany: Plants Affecting Man's Health.* New York: John Wiley and Sons, 1977.

Lloyd, J.U. *Eclectic Med J.* 1897:427.

Lloyd, J.U. *A Treatise on Echinacea.* Drug Treatise No. 30. Cincinnati, OH: Lloyd Brothers, Pharmacists, Inc, 1924.

Luettig. B., Steinmüller, C., Gifford, G.E., Wagner, H., Lohmann-Matthes. "Macrophage activation by the polysaccharide arabinogalactin isolated from plant cell cultures of *Echinacea purpurea.*" *J Nat Cancer Inst* 1989;82(9): 669–675.

Madaus, G. *Lehrbuch der biologischen Heilmittel.* Hildesheim, Germany: Georg Olms Verlag, 1938.

Mahajan, V.M. "Antimycotic activity of different chemicals, chaksine iodide and garlic." *Mykosen* 1983 Feb;26(2):94–9.

Masini, S. "Case study: a side effect of echinacea?" *Medical Herbalism* 1992;4(2):8.

McAnalley, B.H. and McDaniel, H.R. International Patent WO 93/08810 (1993).

McLeod, D. "Case History of Chronic Lymphocytic Leukaemia." *The Modern Phytotherapist* 1996a;2(3):10.

McLeod, D. Personal communication. December, 1996b.

McLeod, D., Bone, K., and Morgan M. "Potential hepatotoxicity in patients receiving herbal medicine in a clinical setting—a preliminary report." *European Journal of Herbal Medicine* 1996;2(3):39–48.

Meissner, H.K.L. "Zur behandlung der chronischer Polyarthritis rheumatica." *Therapiewoche* 1950a;1:452–453.

Meissner, H.K.L. *Medizin Heute* 1950(b) 11:1–3.

Meissner, H.K.L. *Therapiewoche* 1951;9:522–523.

Mengs, U., Clare, C.B., Poiley, J.A. "Toxicity of *Echinacea purpurea.* Acute, subacute, and genotoxicity studies." *Arzneimittelforschung* 1991 Oct;41(10): 1076–81.

Merck Index: Eleventh edition. [Budavari, S., editor.] Rahway, New Jersey: Merck and Company, 1989.

Mili, F., Flanders, W.D., Boring, J.R. et al. "The associations of alcohol drinking and drinking cessation to measures of the immune system in middle-aged men." *Alcohol Clin Exp Res* 1992;16(4):688–94.

Mohan, M., Pant, C.R., Angra, S.K., Manajan, V.M. "Berberine in trachoma." *Indian J Opthalmol* 1982;30:69–75.

Montague, M.W. *High Times* 1986;135:15,83,93.

Moore, G.S., Atkins, R.D. "The fungicidal and fungistatic effects of an aqueous garlic extract on medically important yeast-like fungi." *Mycologia* 1977 Mar–Apr;69(2):341–8.

Moore, M. *Medicinal Plants of the Mountain West.* Santa Fe, NM: Museum of New Mexico Press, 1979.

Moore, M. *Medicinal Plants of the Desert and Canyon West.* Santa Fe, NM: Museum of New Mexico Press, 1989.

Moore, M. *Medicinal Plants of the Pacific West.* Santa Fe, NM; Red Crane Books, 1993.

Moser, J. "Echinacea and a spurious root that appeared in the fall of 1909." *Am J Pharm* 1910;82:224. [Cited in Foster.]

Muller-Jakic, B., Breu, W., Probstle, A., Redl, K., et al. "In vitro inhibition of cyclooxygenase and 5-lipoxygenase by alkamides from Echinacea and Achillea species." *Planta Med* 1994;60(1):37–40.

Mumcuoglu, M. *Sambucus nigra (L), Black Elderberry Extract: A breakthrough in the treatment of influenza.* Skokie, Illinois: RSS Publishing, 1995.

Mund-Hoym W.D. "Wundbehandlung mit echinaceahaltigen Externa." *Arztl. Praxis* 1979;31(14):566–567.

Murphy, R. *Lotus Materia Medica.* Pagosa Springs, CO; Lotus Star Academy, 1995.

Nowak, M.A. and McMichael, A.J. "How HIV Defeats the Immune System." *Scientific American* 1995;273(2);58–65.

Okuyama, E., Umeyama, K., Yamazaki, M., Kinoshita, Y., and Yamamoto, Y. "Usnic acid and diffractaic acid as analgesic and antipyretic components of *Usnea diffracta.*" *Planta Med* 1995;61(2):113–5.

Osol, A. and Farrar, G. *The Dispensatory of the United States of America. 24th Edition*. Philadelphia, Pennsylvania: J.B. Lippencott Company, 1947.

Ostrenga, J.A. and Perry, D. *PharmChem Newsletter* 1975;4(1):1–3.

Parnham, M.J. *Phytomedicine* 1996;3:95–102. Cited in: Bone, K. Phytomedicine Conference Report—Part 2. *MediHerb Monitor* 1996;(November):1.

Pennisi, E. "Food allergies linked to ear infections." *Sci News* 1994;146:231.

Phillips, L.G., Nichols, M.H., King, W.D. "Herbs and HIV: the health food industry's answer." *South Med J.* 1995 Sep;88(9):911–3.

Pizzorno, J. *Total Wellness*. Rocklin, California: Prima Publishing, 1996.

Priest, A.W., and Priest, L.R. *Herbal Medication: A Clinical and Dispensary Handbook*. London: L. N. Fowler and Co, Ltd., 1982.

Proksch, A., and Wagner, H. "Structural analysis of a 4-O-methyl-glucuronoarabinoxylan with immuno-stimulating activity from *Echinncea purpurea*." *Phytochemistry* 1987;26(7):1989–1993.

Qian, H., Dowling, J.E. "Pharmacology of novel GABA receptors found on rod horizontal cells of the white perch retina." *J Neurosci* 1994.

Rabbani, G.H., Butler, T., Knight, J., et al. "Randomized controlled trial of berberine sulfate therapy for diarrhea due to enterotoxigenic *Escherichia coli* and *Vibrio cholerae*." *J Infectious Dis* 1987;155(5):979–984.

Rae, W.J., and Liang, H.C. "Effects of pesticides on the immune system." *J Nutr Med* 2:399–410.

Rafinesque, C.S. *Medical Flora: manual of the medical botany of the United States of America*. Volume 2. Philadelphia: Samuel C. Atkinson, 1830.

Ram, N.H. "Echinacea: Its effect on the normal individual with special reference to changes produced in the blood picture." *Eclectic Medical Journal* 1935; 34–36.

Reuss, D. *Zschr Allg Med* 1979;55(24):1324.

Reuss, D. "Behandlung der chronischen Polyarthritis mit Echinacin." *Rheuma* 1986;5:29–32.

Ringsdorf, W., Cheraskin, E., and Ramsay, R. "Sucrose, neutrophilic phagocytosis and resistance to disease." *Dent Surv* 1976;52:46–48.

Rinkel, H.J., Randolph, T.G., and Zeller, M. *Food Allergy.* Springfield, Illinois: C.C. Thomas, 1951.

Roesler, J., Steinmuller, C., Kiderlen, A., Emmendorffer, A., Wagner, H., Lohmann-Matthes, M.L. "Application of purified polysaccharides from cell cultures of the plant *Echinacea purpurea* to mice mediates protection against systemic infections with *Listeria monocytogenes* and *Candida albicans.*" *Int J Immunopharmacol* 1991;13(1):27–37.

Roesler, J., Emmendorffer, A., Steinmuller, C., Luettig, B., Wagner, H., Lohmann-Matthes, M.L. "Application of purified polysaccharides from cell cultures of the plant *Echinacea purpurea* to test subjects mediates activation of the phagocyte system." *Int J Immunopharmacol* 1991;13(7):931–41.

Sabir, M. Bhide, N.K.. "Study of some pharmacological actions of berberine." *Indian J Physiol Pharmacol* 1971;15:111–132.

Sabir, M., Mahajan, V.M., Mohapatra, L.N., Bhide, N.K. "Experimental study of the antitrachoma action of berberine." *Indian J Med Res* 1976;64:1160–1167.

Sabir, M., Akhter, M.H., and Bhide, N.K. "Antagonism of cholera toxin by berberine in the gastrointestinal tract of adult rats." *Indian J Med Res* 1977;65:305–313.

Sabir, M., Akhter, M.H., and Bhide, N.K. "Further studies on pharmacology of berberine." *Ind J Physiol Pharmacol* 1978;22:9–23.

Sanchez, A., Reeser, J., Lau, H. et al. "Role of sugars in human neutrophilic phagocytosis." *Am J Clin Nutr* 1973;26:1180–1184.

Sandhu, D.K., Warraich, M.K., Singh, S. "Sensitivity of yeasts isolated from cases of vaginitis to aqueous extracts of garlic." *Mykosen* 1980 Dec;23(12): 691–8.

Schimmel, K.Ch. and Werner, G.T. "Nonspecific enhancement of intrinsic resistance to infection by Echinacin." *Ther D Gegenw* 120(11):1065–1076.

Schimmer, O., Abel, G., Behinger, C. "Untersuchungen zur gentoxischen Potenz eines neutralen Polysaccharids aus *Echinacea*-Gewebkulturen in menschliched Lymphozytenkilturen." *Zeitschrift für Phytotherapie* 1989;10:39–42.

Schnursbusch, F. *Z Laryng Rhinol Otol* 1955;34:520.

Schöneberger, D. "The influence of immune-stimulating effects of pressed juice from *Echinacea purpurea* on the course and severity of colds. Results of a double-blind study." *Forum Immunologie* 1992;8:2–12.

Schöpf, J.D. *Materia Medica Americana Potissimum Regni Vegetabilis.* Erlangen, Germany, 1787. Reprinted 1903: Lloyd Library Bulletin No. 6, Reproduction Series No.3, Cincinnati, OH.

Schulte, K.E., Rücher, G., Perlick, J. "Das Vorkommen von Polyacetylen-Verbindungen in *Echinacea purpurea* MOENCH un *Echinacea angustifolia* DC." *Arzneimittel Forschung* 1967;17(7):825–829.

Schuster, A. *Medizinische Monatsschrift* 1952; 7:453–455.

Scudder, J.M. *Specific Medication and Specific Medicines,* Fourth Revision. 15th ed. 1903. Reprinted., Portland OR: Eclectic Medical Publications, 1985.

Sharma, V.D., Sethi, M.S., Kumar, A., Rarotra, J.R. "Antibacterial property of *Allium sativum Linn.*: in vivo & in vitro studies." *Indian J Exp Biol* 1977 Jun;15(6):466–8.

Shashikanth, K.N., Basappa, S.C., Sreenivasa, Murthy, V. "A comparative study of raw garlic extract and tetracycline on caecal microflora and serum proteins of albino rats." *Folia Microbiol (Praha)* 1984;29(4):348–52.

Siegel, R.L., Issekutz, T., Schwabei, J. et al. "Deficiency of T helper cells in transient hypogammaglobulinemia of infancy." *NEJM* 305:1307–1313.

Stansbury, Jill, N.D. Personal communication. Fall, 1994.

Subbaiah, T.V., and Amin, A.H. "Effect of berberine sulfate on *Entamoeba histolytica.*" *Nature* 1967;215;527–528.

Sun, D., Abraham, S.N., Beachey, E.H. "Influence of berberine sulfate on synthesis and expression of Pap fimbrial adhesin in uropathogenic *Escherichia coli.*" *Antimicrob Agents Chemother* 1988;32;1274–1277.

Sun, D. Courtney, H.S., and Beachey, E.H. "Berberine sulfate blocks adherence of streptococcus pyrogenes to epithelial cells, fibronectin and hexadane." *Antimicrob Agents Chemother* 1988;32:1370–1374.

Swabb, E.A., Tai, Y.H., and Jordan, L. "Reversal of cholera toxin-induced secretion in rat ileum by luminal berberine." *Am J Physiol* 1981 Sep;241(3): G248–252.

Tilgner, Dr. Sharol. Personal communication. August, 1996.

Tonnesen, H., Kaiser, A.H., Nielsen, B.B., and Pedersen, A.E. "Reversibility of alcohol-induced immune depression." *Br J Addict* 1992;87(7):1025–8.

Tynecka, Z. and Gos, Z. "The inhibitory action of garlic *(Allium sativum L.)* on growth and respiration of some microorganisms." *Acta Microbiol Pol [B]* 1973;5(1):51–62.

Tynecka, Z. and Gos, Z. "The fungistatic activity of garlic *(Allium sativum L.)* in vitro." *Ann Univ Mariae Curie Sklodowska [Med]* 1975;30:5–13.

Veninga, L., and Zaricor, B.R. *Goldenseal/Etc.* Santa Cruz, California: Ruka Publications, 1976.

Viehmann, P. "Erfahrungen mit einer *Echinacea*-haltigen Hautsalbe." *Erfahrungsheilkunde* 1978;27(6):353–358.

Von Unruh, V. *"Echinacea angustifolia* and *Inula helenium* in the treatment of tuberculosis." *Nat Eclect Med Assoc Quart* 1915;7:63.

Vulto, A.G. and De Smet, P.A.G.M. "Drugs used in non-orthodox medicine." In: Dukes, M.G.N. *Meyler's Side Effects of Drugs,* 11th ed. Amsterdam: Elsevier, 1988.

Wagner, H. and Proksch, A. "Über ein immunostimulierendes Prinzip aus *Echinacea purpurea* MOENCH." *Z für Angew Phytother.* 1981;2:166–171.

Wagner, H. and Proksch, A. "Immunostimulatory drugs of fungi and higher plants." In: *Economic and Medicinal Plant Research,* Vol.1., N. Farnsworth, H.Hikino, and H. Wagner, eds. Orlando, Florida: Academic Press, 1985.

Wagner, H. et al. "Isolation of sesquiterpene derivatives and pharmaceuticals containing these compounds." German patent *(Chem Abstract)* 1987;14(7): 4299–307.

Wagner, H., Stuppner, H., Schäfer, W., and Zenk, M. "Immunologically active polysaccharides of *Echinacea purpurea* cell cultures." *Phytochemistry* 1988; 27(1):119–126.

Wagner, H., Stuppner, H., Puhlmann, J., Brümmer, B., Deppe, K., and Zenk, M.H. "Gewinnung von immunologisch aktiven Polysacchariden aus Echinacea-Drogen und -Gewebkulturen." *Zeitschrift für Phytotherapie* 1989;10: 35–38.

Wagner, H. and Jurcic, K. "Immunologic studies of plant combination preparations. In-vitro and in-vivo studies on the stimulation of phagocytosis." *Arzneimittelforschung* 1991 Oct;41(10):1072–6.

Wei, X., Ghosh, S.K., Taylor, M.E., Johnson, V.A., et al. "Viral dynamics in human immunodeficiency virus type 1 infection." *Nature* 1995 Jan 12; 373(6510):117–22.

Weiss, R.F. *Herbal Medicine*. Beaconsfield, England: Beaconsfield Publishers, 1988. [Translated from the sixth German edition of *Lehrbuch der Phytotherapie* by the same author.]

Werbach, M. *Nutritional Influences on Illness*. Tarzana, California: Third Line Press, 1987.

Willard, T. *The Wild Rose Scientific Herbal*. Calgary, Alberta, Canada: Wild Rose College, 1991.

Wren, C. *Potter's New Cyclopedia of Botanical Drugs and Preparations*. Saffron Walden, England: C.W. Daniel Company, 1989.

Xuan, B., Wang, W., and Li, D.X. "Inhibitory effect of tetrahydroberberine on platelet aggregation and thrombosis." *Chung Kuo Yao Li Hsueh Pao* 1994 Mar;15(2):133–5.

Yamahara, J. "Behavioral pharmacology of berberine-type alkaloids. Central depressive action of *Coptidis rhizoma* and its constituents." *Nippon Yakurigaku Zasshi* 1976 Oct;72(7):899–908. [Japanese language]

Zakay-Rones, Z., Varsano, N., Zlotnik, M., Manor, O., et al. "Inhibition of several strains of influenza virus in vitro and reduction of symptoms by an elderberry extract *(Sambucus nigra* L.) during an outbreak of influenza B in Panama." *Journal of Alternative and Complementary Medicine*. 1995;1(4):361–369.

Zhu, B., and Ahrens, F.A. "Effect of berberine on intestinal secretion mediated by *Escherichia coli* heat-stable enterotoxin in jejunum of pigs." *Am J Vet Res* 1982 Sep;43(9):1594–8.

Zhu, B., and Ahrens, F. "Antisecretory effects of berberine with morphine, clonidine, L-phenylephrine, yohimbine or neostigmine in pig jejunum." *Eur J Pharmacol* 1983 Dec 9;96(1–2):11–9.

INDEX